THE MIRACLES OF URINE-THERAPY

by
Dr. Beatrice Bartnett
and
Margie Adelman, L.M.T., C.N.

DISCLAIMER

The therapy outlined in this book is an entirely drugless system of healing.

The author's believe that the body's innate wisdom has the ability to heal itself. However, as of this printing, the legal system states that only M.D.'s may claim cures. Therefore, the authors do not recommend that anyone follows this procedure unless they consult their physician beforehand.

©1987 by Dr. Beatrice Bartnett and
Margie Adelman.
All rights reserved.
ISBN: 0-9619997-0-5

No part of this book may be reproduced or utilized in any form or by any means, electronical or mechanical, including photocopying, recording, or by any information storage and retrieval system, without permission in writing from both authors. It may not be translated in any other language without expressed written consent from both authors.

Cover design:
1987 Turk Winterrowd, New York.

First printed edition 1987
Manufactured in the United States of America.

DEDICATION

This book is dedicated to all persons who are suffering from dis-ease, mainly the AIDS patients. May they heal themselves and Mother Earth — and bring peace to Mankind.

ACKNOWLEDGEMENTS

A special thanks to my husband Dr. Edmond R. Bartnett for his emotional and financial support, without him this book would not have been possible.

Thanks to our brother Mark, who made our encounter possible, and for opening his home to us to let this wonderous work flow through.

We would also like to thank Bejamin Franklin for his guidance, and send him a red rose. Thank you Ben!

Most of all, we would like to thanks our parents, Peter and Claudette Rotella, and Paul and Margaritha Nellen, for the opportunity to be alive and for their love.

A special thanks to the Rotella clan for their love and continued support: Tommy, Elaine, Debbie, Claudette and Jennifer.

We would like to acknowledge the following people for their support:

June Bartnett	*Bernard Schmit*
Alan Burns	*Martin Segal*
Georges and Hildegard Fontana	*Michael Weinstock*
Michelle Newman	*W.T.*
Reverend Inquisitor	*Joy Adelman*

We would like to express deep gratitude to Turk Winterrowd for the cover illustration.

DEFINITION OF UROPATHY

Let it be known that the terms UROPATHY and urine-therapy are used interchangeably throughout this entire book. The word UROPATHY cannot yet be found in the English dictionary. It was fabricated by ME NEW MAN and derived from the words urine *(uro)* and pathy *(dis-ease)*. UROPATHY is the method of healing dis-ease by the application of one's own urine (auto-urine-therapy).

SIGNIFICANCE OF THE BUTTERFLY

The butterfly on the cover has a special symbolic meaning. When the caterpillar enters the cocoon, all of the organs and tissues of its body are reduced to a common fluid. The germ of the butterfly, which is implanted in the caterpillar, is gestated, reshaped, and reborn in the living fluid or water of the cocoon.

When the butterfly emerges from its baptismal ceremony, it is a reborn being: it is a transformed being: it is a new being: it is possessed of superior powers and, through its glorious transformation, it is adapted to a new and superior plane of life.

ABOUT THE AUTHORS

Dr. Beatrice Bartnett - was born and raised in Switzerland. She studied Naturopathy in Freiburg, Germany, and practiced in Switzerland as a Naturopathic Physician. She gave lectures and wrote numerous articles pertaining to holistic medicine. She wrote her first book on Shiatsu, and taught differtent aspects of bodywork.

In 1985 Dr. Bartnett completed her studies as a Chiropractic Physician at the Life Chiropractic College in Georgia. After practicing in the States as a Chiropractor, she returned to Switzerland, where she was exposed to many spiritual healing methods including UROPATHY. She followed this path and is now lecturing, giving seminars and private consultations all over the world.

Margie Adelman, L.M.T., C.N. -was born in 1960 in Huntington, New York. She completed High School in Oxon Hill. Maryland. In Los Angeles, California she studied nutrition. In 1984 she attended the Palm Beach School for Holistic Massage and became a Licensed Massage Therapist. She worked with a Naturopathic Physician administering colonics and composing herbal remedies.

She has presently given up a very successful private massage practice to dedicate her life to healing with UROPATHY. She cured herself of Hypoglycemia using this method. After four years of extensive research on UROPATHY she is holding seminars and giving private consultations worldwide.

FOREWARD

How fortunate you are to be alive in this great time; in this time of change and growth. Mankind is growing from adolescence into adulthood, and you will help this process.

Give thanks that you are one of the chosen ones to be alive in this special hour. Listen to the voice inside you, so that you will fulfill your destiny and the destiny of Mankind, Mother Earth, and the Universe.

This is the time the prophets foretold in their books. Mankind has been waiting thousands of years for its arrival and you are a part of it.

Love yourself, you are very special. Love will move mountains, heal the sick and develop the arts and sciences.

Love yourself for what you are, a God or Goddess — perfect, loving, and good.

The Water of Life is a gift given by your creator for your spiritual growth and physical well-being.

It was used by the spiritual leaders, sacred groups, and simple folk through all ages.

It was never lost, only hidden, for truth always exists.

You were guided to find this information, read it and meditate it. Let God within be your teacher and go over those obstacles which may hinder you on your path. Ask for guidance and it shall be given to you.

Give thanks to be a part of this wondrous plan!

But most of all —love yourself— love will move any atoms in the universe and bring positive changes to these times.

With love,
Margie Adelman
Dr. Beatrice Bartnett

TABLE OF CONTENTS

	Introduction	1
Chapter 1	Metaphysical History of Uropathy	5
Chapter 2	Science and Uropathy	15
Chapter 3	Aids and Uropathy	21
Chapter 4	How to use Uropathy (treatment)	29
Chapter 5	Reactions to Uropathy	35
Chapter 6	Herbs and Vitamins	39
Chapter 7	Healthy Lifestyle	45
Chapter 8	Holistic Healing	51
Chapter 9	Our-Self-Involvement	55
Chapter 10	Case Histories and Testimonials	61
Chapter 11	Conclusion	75
	List of Suggested Resources	82
	Bibliography	84

INTRODUCTION

This book has been written to expose the truth.

We have reached a time, when people must become responsible for their own health-care.

The close rapport between physician and patient has been deteriorating for quite some time. Intelligent members of the public are growing more distrustful of orthodox medical treatments.

We believe that the medical establishment is partially responsible for limiting their research, after proving the efficacy of urine in the treatment of certain dis-eases, one being cancer.

The research on this topic has been very limited due to the fact that it is not a profitable means of healing.

We do not make claims for any cures, we are only following the policy required from all reputable members of the medical profession themselves, to make no secret of any discovery which may prove useful in helping mankind.

Many people believe that thousands of doctors, vast hospitals, an overabundance of nurses, dentists, chemists, and clinics are signs of progressive medical abilities, when actually they demostrate failure of our medical system. Contributing to this is wrong guidance of the public in nutrition and other ways of living.

Thousands of operations performed weekly with brilliant technique prove only further that prior treatments had not achieved a successful cure.

Many people must have asked themselves the following questions:

1) Why can nothing better than the knife, radiation or chemotherapy be suggested after 50 years of orthodox cancer research?

2) Why is it that when effective treatments for cancer or other dis-eases have been discovered either by a qualified doctor, or by practitioners of an unorthodox school, they have not been recognized by the cancer association or any other related organizations, which still asks the public to donate large sums of money toward the discovery of a cure?

There are no satisfactory answers!

We do not wish to do injustice to those unselfish and honest physicians who are practicing what they really believe in. Caring doctors are urgently needed. Many of these health praticioners are putting their licences on the line by helping other people. Others have left the country so they can practice medicine in a more natural, humanistic and effective way.

We have no patent or medicine to sell. UROPATHY can be carried out at home without any financial outlay whatsoever.

We make no claims of having a cure, we only read scientific studies, case histories, and metaphysical literature, which is pointing in that direction.

The doctor of the future will be a teacher, and the patients will be the healers. The doctor will educate the people on how to take care of themselves on a physical, emotional and spiritual level. The patient will spend more time and interest on how the body functions, how to take care of it, the meaning of life and the resposibilities toward himself/herself and society.

The world is in the midst of major changes. The biggest challenge will be to take responsibility of one's life into one's own hands. This will not be an easy process and it requires time —time for learning.

Many people are already on their way to holostic living, and many more will follow. The next generation, and the generations to come will be better prepared, stronger and healthier in every way.

We would like to close this introduction with some quoted opinions from two doctors about UROPATHY.

Dr. N. Mehta, M.D. (London). Former Chief Minister of Gujarat, writes in his forward to the book "Manav Mootra" (English Edition) — *"The belief that urine is not an excreta, but is an elixir of life, gifted by nature for the purpose of healthy living and for use as a main therapeutic measure for almost the whole range of human diseases including Cancer, T.B., Leprocy, etc., is intriguing, interesting, and fascinating. If it could be substantiated by human experiments undertaken and planned on a scientific basis, it would be a great boon to human beings, more so in the modern age of space travel."*

Dr. P.D. Desai, M.B.B.S., states: *"The fact that auto-urine provides a universal remedy for curing the patients' illnesses of every kind, including Cancer, Heart disease, Diabetes, T.B., Leprocy, etc., is amply proved during the past 60 years by innumerable clinical tests conducted in the U.S.S.R., Italy, France, Germany, India, etc. But we allopaths generally fight shy in accepting new trends in medical treatment, unless clinical trials prove their efficacy. Even then medical opinion may come to be divided. It has been demonstrated by certain "Big Wigs" in the medical profession by very risky experiments made on their ownselves, that 'MOST DEADLY BACTERIA ARE HARMLESS IN A HEALTHY BODY.' As found in the scientific researches conducted in the U.S.A., Japan, etc., human urine contains various hormones, enzymes, vitamins, antibodies, antigens, salts, etc. It is therefore no wonder if the treatment with auto-urine which contains such valuable substances, makes the sick body healthy by stimulating its vital force —the defense mechanism of the body, and makes it IMMUNE to the most deadly bacteria, viruses, toxins, etc. and cures illnesses of all kinds."*

METHAPHYSICAL HISTORY
OF
UROPATHY

The supporting metaphysical evidence and history of UROPATHY is so vast and profuse that we cannot elaborate in one such publication. A second publication directed toward the philosophical and historical background of this topic is forthcoming.

In this chapter, it is our intention to briefly discuss the relativity of UROPATHY to the major religions of the world and other sacred groups, uniting all the different faiths bound by common truth for peace and harmony to reside over the planet.

If you seek to expand your knowledge through back-up research on this topic, please keep in mind that urine is synonomous and interchangeable with the following terms and phrases: Tree of Life, Manna, Soma, Blood of Christ, Blood of the Lamb, Living Waters, Elixir, Water of Life, Bodily Fluids, River of Life, Lotus Flower, Rose, Cross, Ankh, Wine, Spring, Well, Stream, Fountain of Life, Fountain of Youth, and others.

Extensive research into metaphysical books, the bible, and books listed in the bibliography can be used as references to confirm and legitimize these claims. You will begin to see that the pieces of the puzzle start to fit together.

Drinking the "Waters" of your body is not something new. It was used since the beginning of time. Through our research we found overwhelming metaphysical evidence supporting UROPATHY.

The truth never died; it has only been hidden, and this is the truth, my friends.

This therapy has been passed down from ancient civilizations, religious sacred groups, and even Jesus spoke about it.

Authentic documents that have been unveiled possess powerful significant symbols used for communication amongst these ancient cultures. The Egyptian hieroglyphics, sanskrit, and many other pictorial symbols were used to keep the truth hidden from the profane and ignorant.

Over the centuries, people came to regard their bodies as filthy and shameful organisms. People lost touch with their divinity and the perfection of their own creation. Those of you who say you believe in God, whoever your God is, do you really think that our all-loving omnipotent Creator would have created such injustice as dis-ease? No, my friends, we have manifested our own injustice and dis-ease. It is now time for us to come to this realization.

All through the Bible one can find many references concerning the "Water of Life", which man has interpreted a thousand different ways to avoid hearing the truth.

In the Old Testament we find, *"Drink thy waters of thine own cistern, and running waters from your own well."* **(Proverb 5:15)**, and *"For the whole house of Ahab shall perish; and I will cut off from Ahab him that pisseth against the wall, and him that is shut up and left in Israel."* **(II Kings 9:8)**.

In the New Testament Jesus spoke many times about drinking the "Water of Life." In the book of John we found passages such as this, *"Out of his belly shall flow rivers of living water,"* **(John 7:38)**. Do you really think he meant anything other than what these statements literally imply. It is true that for the most part the Bible was written in symbols and parables, but there are a few very direct veritable passages that man in all his ignorance cannot escape, such as this one: *"But whoever drinks of the water that I shall give him will never thirst. But the water that I shall give him will become in him a fountain of water springing up into everlasting life."* ***(John 4:14)***. With deeper research we found that the blood of Jesus was a similitude for the "Water of Life." In many books about the Great White Brotherhood, Masons, and the Rosicrucians, we found several indications to the drinking of the "Water of Life."

In India, the yogi's and the great spiritual masters were well aware of the miracles of this sacred fluid. Gandhi drank his urine daily and survived long periods of fasting on it. The American and South American Indians are also well informed of the efficacy of urine and consider it a perfect elixir for the functioning of healthy bodies as well as a tincture for healing the sick and dis-eased.

Taking into consideration that these people knew all along about UROPATHY and used it as part of their daily regime, why is it so difficult for our society to accept something that has been innate wisdom for centuries?

A possible answer to this question is shame of the human body, originating from the concept of Adam and Eve. Writings from the Gospel of Philip taken from Christian Texts and New Testament Apochrypha state, *"When Eve was in Adam, there was no death; but when she was separated from him death came into being. If she returns unto him, death will no longer exist."*

It was not until they disobeyed the Lord by eating the forbidden fruit, that they were cast out of paradise and became aware of the darkness, evil, and their naked bodies.

This separation of man and woman marked the beginning of death and division of the sexes. Christ came in order that he might remove the separation and again unite the two: and that he might give life to those who died in the separation and unite them.

By drinking the "Water of Life" man can restore a state of androgeny and regain the true meaning behind his/her creation. This occurs through purification of the body, mind, and spirit. This process is called "transmutation."

Albert Einstein proved that matter and energy are interchangeable. Matter is the physical body, and energy is the spiritual soul. By smashing an atom, energy is released. By applying physical principles, spirituality is obtained.

This rejuvenation alters the vibratory rate of the body and sets in motion the interchange from matter to energy. This is the "transmutation" of the body into spiritual form, called the resurrection.

By not drinking this water and eating earthly foods, these vibrations can be slowed down to the gross material forms we now inhabit. The Old Testament says, "They have forsaken the Fount of Living Waters. We now live in the wake of that rebellion."

Jewish Texts and Old Testament Apochrypha are also filled with similar evidence to the drinking of one's own urine: The First Book of Adam and Eve, Secrets of Enoch, Odes of Solomon, Second Book of Esdras, Fragments of a Zadokite Work, Testament of the Twelve Patriarchs, Book of Judith, Midrash of the Song of Songs of Solomon, and the Dead Sea Scrolls contain an abundance of passages relating to the "Water of Life". However, one must keep in mind that any of the previously mentioned synonymous terms may have been used.

The Dead Sea Scrolls were discovered in 1947, by an Arab shepard in a cave at the Northwestern end of the Dead Sea. In 1949, scholars and archeologists admitted authenticity of the scrolls. The Essenes were the true owners of the scrolls, and what gave the Essenes their peculiar interest to religious historians was the possibility that their kind of Judaism might have served as the matrix for that even more unorthodox Jewish faith we call Christianity. Of all the recorded varieties of Judaism, that of the Essenes, as far as it was known, seemed closest to the religion of the New Testament. Whatever the differences between the Dead Sea Scrolls and the New Testament in their understanding of the messianic office, they clearly share a common Jewish background and find their support in the same profhetic texts of the Old Testament.

The following quotes are taken from the Dead Sea Scrolls. ***(Revelation 22-1-2)*** *"Then he showed me the river of the water of life, bright as a crystal, flowing from the throne of God and the lamb, through the middle of the street of the city; also on either side of the river, the Tree of Life with its twelve kinds of fruits, yielding its fruit each month; and the leaves of the tree were for the healing of the nation."*

> *"I (thank Thee, O Lord, for) Thou hast lodged me beside*
> *a fountain of running waters in a waterless land,*
> *and by a spring in a parched land,*
> *and by channels that irrigate a garden (of delight in the wilderness.)*
>
> *But Thou, O my God, hast put into my mouth*
> *as showers of early rain for all (those who thirst)*
> *and a spring of living water..."*.
>
> ***(Hymns, Col. VIII)***

In the Hindu Sastra we found in ***Verse VI. (1:3 Hyms of the Artharvaveda)*** contained passages such as this:

"The waters verily are healing. The waters chase away dis-ease, the waters cure all (dis-ease): may they prepare a remedy for thee!" ***Verse II. 9:5*** *— "The god (man) that has caused (dis-ease) shall perform the cure, he is himself the best physician."* ***Verse VI 85:1, 3*** *— "This divine tree, the varana, shall shut out (dis-ease). As vritra did hold fast these ever-flowing waters, thus do I shut out dis-ease from thee with (the help of) Agni Vaisvanara."*

Most of the yogi's and eastern spiritual masters of our time are fully aware of the powers of urine, but were sworn to secrecy, keeping the truth hidden, so that they could be praised and worshipped as Gods by their people. This was indeed a selfish act and has caused much suffering and unnecessary deaths for the mere enjoyment of ego.

In Buddhist and Taoist Texts we discovered youth and beauty associated with bodily fluids. In the Hevajra Tantra, verses such as this appear: *"He should always eat herbs and drink water, then old age and death will not harm him, and he will always be protected"*.

The next verse is taken from, The Legend of the Great Stupa, which is also part of the Buddhist and Taoist Texts. *"... Whoever offers food for the sacrament obtains supreme realization and spiritual powers, and all potential arising in the mind will become actual: whoever offers water perfumed with the five scents has his darkness illuminated and is reborn with nobility and attractive purity."*

The Sufi Texts of the Islam states:

Verse XXXV

*Then to the lip of this poor earthen
Urn
I lean'd the Secret of my life to learn.
And lip to lip it murmur'd —
"While you live.
Drink! —for, once dead, you never
shall return."*

Verse XXXVI

*I think the Vessel, that with fugitive
Articulation answer'd, once did live.
And drink: and Ah! the passive lip
I kiss'd
How many Kisses might it take —and
give!*

Verse XXXIX

*And not a drop that from our Cups
we throw
For Earth to drink of, but may steal
below
To quench the fire of Anguish in
some Eye
There hidden —far beneath, and long
ago.*

Baha'u'llah writes in The Hidden Words, a scripture from the Baha'i faith, the following:

"O SON OF DUST! Turn not away from the matchless wine of the immortal Beloved, and open them not to foul and immortal dregs. Take from the hands of the divine

Cup-bearer the chalice of immortal life, that all wisdom may be thine, and that thou mayest hearken unto the mystic voice calling from the realm of the invisible. Cry aloud, ye that are of low aim! Wherefore have ye turned away from My holy and immortal wine unto evanescent water?"

"O SON OF MAN! A dewdrop out of the fathomless ocean of My mercy I have shed upon the peoples of the world, yet found none turn thereunto, inasmuch as everyone hath turned away from the celestial wine of unity into the foul dregs of impurity, and content with mortal cup, hath put away the chalice of immortal beauty. Vile is that wherewith he is contented."

Other sacred groups including the Masons, Rosicrucians, and the Universal White Brotherhood possess secret documents containing the rituals and doctrines that drinking one's own urine is very efficacious in purifying the body of all poisonous matter. It also gives eternal youth and vibrant health.

In a book written by Omraam Mikhael Aivanhov, called the "Mysteries of Yesod", about the initiatic teachings of the Universal White Brotherhood, are a plethora of quotes directly stating the benefits of drinking one's own urine.

Suppose you wish to purify yourself where there is no water. Imagine a feeling of freshness, as if drops of water were falling on you and carrying off all your impurity. This spiritual bath is most effective because as I have said, the real water is not physical, inside man is a spring of living water, and that is what Jesus meant when he said, 'From his belly shall flow rivers of living water. .' Physical water is nothing but a means of communication with the spiritual water."

Another quote reads: *"We have seen that life is a current, a river that comes from the heights, from the Spring: The River of Life is the Christ. That is why Jesus said, 'I am the way the truth and the life.' An initiatic hearing those words has before him a mental image of a river coursing down the mountainside and melting into the sea. The way, the truth, and the life, what do those words signify? The way is the riverbed, life is the water that flows along the riverbed, the truth is the spring, the beginning of everything, from which life and all creatures come."*

Still another reads: *"Water is the symbol of love: the energies and forces circulating in nature and the cosmos are the fluid, the water that quenches and restores life."*

A quote from the works of the Rosicrucian Brotherhood states: *"And God has promised through his prophets, in the last days before the end of the world, 'to pour out His spirit upon all flesh' **(Joel 2:28),** and the royal psalmist prophecies that God will quench the thirst of the sons of men out of the stream of His grace: Those who remain under the protection of his wings in hope will find in him the fountain of life for in his light we shall see the light."*

Indian legends abound with accounts of the bearded man who spoke a thousand languages and could do anything. He was called Chee-soos, and was known as the serpent (water) God. He was called many names such as Wake, and Quetzalcoatl. The ancient Mayan scriptures, Popol Vuh, further verify these accounts. Even to this day the Zuni Indians of New Mexico perform the sacred ritual of drinking the urine.

Sadly enough the Indians, as well as the religious groups mentioned, were forced to adopt other religions and customs as white man and the churches came in and took over. Their old customs and rituals soon died out and were lost, nevertheless, the documented proof still exists. The truth remained in secrecy amongst elected individuals by the wise old survivors. That was how it was kept alive up until today.

The Masonic teachings have come to be called the Lost Word, but they have no one to blame but themselves for this loss. Carnal man's common jealously and dislike for spiritual things are the key motivators in the destruction of the True Gospel and negative reception for its teachers. *"To him that overcometh will I give to eat of the hidden manna."* **(Revelation 2:17).**

Other reasons for the loss of this doctrine is the burning of libraries containing scriptures and writings of Jesus, ordered by the Kings and Emperors centuries after his death.

Many of the teachings purporting the benefits derived from urine as part of a daily ritual were destroyed. The only ones with the knowledge kept it a secret for fear of their lives if they were caught teaching it.

The True Gospel was not always a secret. It was once common knowledge and was taught to children from their very birth. The fact that it is now secret is not by divine decree but is the result of increasing evil in the world.

Fear of psychic experience is another reason why they rationalized that the truth must be hidden. In seeking to hide the truth from others, we destroy it under the guise of protecting it.

People became egotistical with their complex intellectual learning. This egotism prevents even such elementary laws as UROPATHY from being understood by them. For how can it profit you if you know many things but do not know yourself? We tell you, friends, man's intellect will be the cause of his own demise!

To those of you who wish to be healed, there is healing; for those of you who turn your heads from the truth there is no mercy!

The time is drawing near; we are in the midst of the prophecies. It is happening now. Please look deep within your souls for the answers; the choice is up to you!

*"Ask, and it will be given to you; seek, and you will find; knock, and it will be opened to you. For everyone who asks receives, and he who seeks finds, and to him who knocks it will be opened." **(Matthew 7:7-8)***

Here are some other Verses in the Bible which have shrouded the truth over the ages.

• *And He said unto me... I am Alpha and Omega, the beginning and the end. I will give unto him that is amidst of the fountain of the water of life freely.* ***(Revelation 21:6)***

• *For My people have committed two evils; they have forsaken Me the fountain of living waters, and hewed them out cisterns, broken cisterns, that can hold no water.* ***(Jer. 2:13)***

• *Be to Me as a resevoir where I can store up My reserve of strength and power and blessing, and make it readily available to the thirsty. (**Luke 11:6**)*

• *Take from me largely, that ye be never holding an empty cup when the thirsty ask of thee a drink, and be never lacking when the sick ask for bread. (**Mark 7:27**)*

• *Receive of My love freely. Drink of My Spirit yea, drink deeply, so that it shall be truly waters to swim in. (**Ezek. 45:5**)*

• *And the Lord shall guide thee continually, and satisfy thy soul in drought, and make fat thy bones: and thou shalt be like a watered garden, and like a spring of water, whose waters fail not. (**Isa. 58:11**)*

SCIENCE AND UROPATHY

Drinking one's own urine may be quite controversial until its value has been experienced personally.

Let us look at some common questions. Many people believe that urine is a toxic substance. If this belief were true, how could anyone survive on urine when they are trapped in a life boat or raft for weeks, or when they are lost in the desert for days? The governments of several countries recommend to their soldiers to drink their own urine in cases of liquid shortage —would they really poison their own people?

There are many persons alive and healthy that are drinking their urine daily. Some have been doing it for over ten years. We also have to consider that what may act as a toxin outside of its natural environment, may not act as a toxin in its own natural environment. The scientific community has spoken of the substances contained in urine which are efficacious in fighting fungal, bacterial, and viral infections. These statements denounce the belief that urine is a toxic or poisonous substance.

One might say, "We should not give back to the body what the body expells." Look and learn from nature. The leaves fall from the trees in autumn. They nourish the ground, which in turn will nourish the tree's roots. Dead leaves are one of the best composts which will produce beautiful, healthy flowers, and trees with excellent fruit.

Another example would be Mother Earth's own water cycle. The sun picks up water from the ocean and creates clouds which cause rain. These rains nurture the grounds, plants, trees, animals and humans. The water flows back into the ocean, where the cycle will begin all over again.

Nature produces everything for a reason; nothing is wasted. A lesson for our society to learn. What Mother Earth produces is returned to her. This is a healthy recycling of matter.

It is very similar with our bodies. The scientific evaluation of urine confirms this principle. Urine is an exact hologram of a healthy or dis-eased body and contains the exact combination of substances the body needs at that time. Let us take a look at these substances.

Urine composition taken from Taber's Encyclopedic Medical Dictionary 13th Edition.

Water 95%
Solids 5%

ORGANIC SUBSTANCES
Urea
Uric Acid
Creatine
Creatinine
Ammonia

INORGANIC SUBSTANCES
Sodium Chloride
Potassium Chloride
Calcium
Magnesium
Phosphorus

It also contains: carbohydrates, pigments, fatty acids, carbonates, bicarbonates, carbonic acid, mucin, mucin-like substances, enzymes, hormones, vitamins, aminoacids, antibodies, minerals and antigens.

Antibody activity in urine has been demonstrated against several micro-organisms. Several authors have reported antibody activity against various bacteria and viruses.

Kurt Herz and Johann Abelle, both M.D.'s used UROPA-

THY very successfully with their patients. They recommended urine for the following dis-eases:
- Any dis-ease related to spastic muscle problems (bronchi, arteries, or uterus)
- Viral and bacterial infections
- Allergies
- Pregnancy problems

During our research on UROPATHY, we discovered some very remarkable studies. Most have been conducted in England and the USA.

Professor John W. Plesch, M.D. did a study on UROPATHY in the 1940's. In his paper he states, "Since I started autourine therapy three years ago, I have not come across a single case where the patient suffered any harm. It is for this reason that I decided to publish my findings at this early stage. The observations are without a doubt sufficient to indicate to the expert that a completely new field of research is being opened up to our knowledge of bacteriology, immunology, and serology. A first step in this direction will obviously be the examination from a immunological point of view of the substances secreted in the urine in the course of the various infectious diseases."

Unfortunately, in a world of modern medicine and pharmaceutical interests, a tincture free and self-produced, will not profit the health industry. For this reason, a very limited amount of research has been done on this topic.

In the 1940's, when John Armstrong, Dr. Herz and Dr. Abelle were writing their books, they shared the common philosophy that antibodies were present in the urine. At that time there was no scientific evidence supporting their beliefs. Therefore, our first step was to look for any scientific studies, or research conducted to prove their theories. Bingo! — "Characterization of Antibodies in Human Urine," a study done by Lars. A. Hanson and Eng M. Tan at the Rockefeller Institute, New York in 1965 showed antibodies for Cholera, Salmonella typhi, Diphtheria, Tetanus toxoid, and Polio present in human urine.

In 1966 M.W. Turner and D.S. Rowe at the Department of

Experimental Pathology, University of Birmingham, finished a study on the "Antibodies of IgA and IgG class in Normal Urine."

During the same year Dr. Merler studied the property of isolated serum and urinary antibodies to a single antigen.

John W. Armstrong treated thousand of patients. He was very successful with the application of UROPATHY against several dis-eases such as Cancer, Allergies, Malaria, Cholera, etc.

In 1973 Dr. Desai, Chief Medical Officer of Bulsar, India concurred with S.L. Jamison about Dr. Simmieons who worked in Italy with obesity and developed certain theories.

Dr. Simmieons postulated that the fundamental mechanism in obesity was due to the malfunction of the diencephalon, and this postulate is supported by facts. There are many obese people who maintain their weight on starvation diets, so the fundamental mechanism has to be something other than excessive intake of calories.

Dr. Desai found that urine contains an as yet unidentified hormone which produces the same results as Dr. Simmieons injections of the synthetically manufactured hormone called chorionic gonadotropin, which he used very successfully in his obesity therapy.

Dr. Desai has stated that "I went on autogenous urine therapy and noticed the same thing. It simply melts like magic." It is believed this is due to the regulation of the diencephalon. The driving desired to eat is not there. Several people lost weight with UROPATHY even though there was no loss of appetite, or changes in their calorie intake.

In 1983 C.W.M. Wilson and A. Lewis did a study on "Auto-Immune Therapy against Human Allergic Disease: A Physiological Self Defense Factor." They wrote, "Guinea pigs sensitized to ovalbumen excrete the antigen in their urine in a therapeutic concentration which prevents anaphylactic death after injection of a challenge dose of the ovalbumen. Sublingual administration of the correct dose of urine from allergic patients also provides therapeutic control of their allergic symptoms." Furthermore they wrote, "Auto-immune buccal urine therapy (AIBUT) is capable of controlling a wide range of blood extrinsic and chemical sensitivity."

In 1984 C.W.M. Wilson did another study on the protective effect of AIBUT against Raynaud Phenomenon. This time the question to be answered was not the efficacy of AIBUT but rather the proper dosage of sublingual administration.

Wilson also found that there was no effect with boiled urine. He saw that the substances in the urine had to be alive and fresh to be used successfully.

The body in its own infinite wisdom produces this perfect substance, not for us to take what we perceive as useful, but to use it as a complete whole serum tincture. The way urine is produced, is how it must be absorbed. The body does not need mind intervention. Just let it do its job, and support it with a very healthy, wholesome diet.

AIDS AND UROPATHY

Acquired Inmmune Deficiency Syndrome appears to be the new killer dis-ease of this century. Fortunately, things are not always as they appear.

AIDS is merely an expression of our lifestyle and philosophies. Viruses were and always have been around or within us. In a healthy body these micro-organisms are not necessarily damaging.

Did you ever ask yourself why certain children contracted Polio and others did not? Why certain people get flus and colds and others do not? Why only 20-30% of the people exposed to the AIDS-virus will manifest fullblown AIDS?

When one has an Acquired Immune Deficiency then the body is vulnerable to many different kinds of infections and dis-eases. Let us look at some of the major infections associated with AIDS:

VIRAL INFECTIONS:	Cytomegalovirus (CMV), Epstein Barr Virus (EBV), Herpes Simplex I and II, Varicella Zoster (Chickenpox, Shingles), Hepatitis, Adenovirus, HTLV-III/LAV (AIDS-Virus).
PARASITIC INFECTIONS:	Pneumocystic carinii pneumonia (PCP), Toxoplasmosis, Amebiasis, Giardiasis, Cryptosporidiosis.
BACTERIAL INFECTIONS:	Tuberculosis, Atypical Tuberculosis, Salmonellosis, Norcardia Infections, Listeria Infections.
FUNGAL INFECTIONS:	Candida Albicans, Cruptococcus, Histoplasma.
BLOOD DISORDERS:	Pancytopenia, Immune Thrombocytopenis Purpura.
CANCER:	Kaposi's Sarcoma, Non-Hodgkin's Disease, Burkitt's Lymphoma, Cancer of the Oropharynx (mouth), Hepatocellular Cancer (liver), Chronic Lymphocytic Leukemia, Lung Cancer (Adenosquamous Type).

It is not necessary to go into details of the AIDS-symptoms and diagnosis. There are already publications which explain all this up to date. Our interest is showing the readers possible causes as well as options and choices for treatment, so one can take their health into their own hands. Ultimately one is responsible for his/her own life, health, happiness, success and peace.

There are several hypothetical causes of AIDS. One of them is that AIDS is caused by a virus called HTVL-III/LAV (Human T-Lymphotropic Virus/ Lymphadenopathy-associated Virus). This virus can be found in **almost all** AIDS-patients. It is also believed that many other micro-organisms play a role in the cause of AIDS.

The AIDS virus according to some scientists may be a metamorphic organism. This is a microbe that changes forms. In the case of AIDS it may express itself as a bacteria, virus, fungi or protozoa. The microbe can change its form at anytime.

Dr. Alan Cantwell, an AIDS-researcher noted that some AIDS patients do not have the famous AIDS virus in their blood. Dr. Cantwell writes in his book, "Aids — The Mystery and the Solution", that "Bacteria... have never been seriously considered as primary causative agents in AIDS. Scientists simply do not believe that bacteria causes chronic diseases, such as AIDS and Cancer. The denial of bacteria in AIDS was due to the century old assumption that bacteria could never be implicated in any form of Cancer. My belief, based on research studies, is that AIDS is Cancer, and Cancer is AIDS. One possible reason for the emergency of the new epidemic of AIDS is that medical scientists may have unwittingly produced more virulent and more contagious cancer bacteria (or viruses), by the widespread use of chemotherapy, antibiotic therapy, and radioactive therapy, in the modern treatment of Cancer."

Dr. Robert Gallo of the National Cancer Institute, who discovered the AIDS virus is opposed to the pleomorphic microbe theory. He calls it insanity. In the meantime millions of dollars continue being spent on AIDS research and treatment sanctioned by Gallo and his supporters, while the alternative AIDS research is being ignored.

With this in mind, we would like to share two articles related to Cancer and UROPATHY. "Chemicals from Urine Changes Cancer Cells." Annheim, California —(AP) "A chemical with the power to change cancer cells back to normal cells has been extracted from human urine and may explain why some cases of Cancer cure themselves, a Baylor University researcher says."

"If the naturally-occuring substance can be made artificially," Dr. S.R. Burzynski said, "it could be valuable in cancer therapy because it does not seem to affect normal cells."

A report presented at the annual meeting of the "Federation of American Society for Experimental Biology," in Atlantic City, USA in April 1966 under the heading, "Bringing Cancer Cells into Line," gives the account of research showing the effect of human urine in cancer cells..." The two researchers found unexpectedly that the urine extract, which they called 'Directin' when added to the culture medium causes all the cancer cells on which it has so far been tested, to align themselves end-to-end into straight rows..."

Successful results have been demonstrated by many cancer patients who recovered using UROPATHY. Current studies with UROPATHY and AIDS show promising results. Because of the nature of this dis-ease, the studies in progress will require long term observation.

Why are micro-organisms able to easily take over our immune system? These parasites called viruses, bacteria, fungi, and protozoa habitate and flourish in our bodies, because of the provided environment established by our unhealthy lifestyles.

We do not believe that AIDS is a NEW virus. The most important answer for prevention and cure of AIDS should be directed toward strengthening the body, in a physical, emotional and spiritual way, as well as cleaning up our living environment especially our air and water.

AIDS is only one expression of decreased vitality, there is also an increase in T.B., Syphilis and other infections as well as chronic dis-eases. Even though medical standards are very high, there are more dis-eased children today than ever before. It appears in general that immune systems are weaker, and people are an easier target for any dis-ease.

The main contributor to the problem of dise-ease is our eating habits. We now have the third generation on junk-foods, soft drinks, and artificial additives. These substances are not only useless for our bodies in terms of nutrients; they are harmful. The body can fight only so much and so long. These weakened bodies are giving birth to children. How strong and healthy do you think these babies will be? The long term effects are just beginning to surface. Only this time it will not appear in guinea pigs, no, this time it appears in people, — you and me.

Another factor contributing to the cause of dis-ease is immunization. Immunization decreases the body's ability to remain healthy. The body has a built-in immune system. This system has taken care of civilization for thousands of years. It was not vaccines, drugs, antibiotics or operations that saved mankind for thousands of years; these methods were unknown until the last two centuries. It was the body's own infinite wisdom, proper nutrition, clean sanitation and avoidance of poisons, that perpetuated a healthy species.

Drinking the Water of Life is only one aspect of the healing process. In order to express optimum health, harmony between the spiritual, emotional, and physical realms must exist.

The prevalence of AIDS appears to be in a time when traditional bonds between families, friends, and even communities are deteriorating. Our lives seem to be moving at a rapid pace and the integral trusting relationships are vanishing.

People on the outskirts of society are more vulnerable to dis-ease because of the increased stress level in their daily lives, and also because of their constant fight for their rights and moral existence.

Let us take a look at the reasons why AIDS is so prevalent in the gay population.

The gay population in the USA is the only minority group which is not yet recognized by the government. Being gay in this society brings one on the edge of a "normal" social life. Either they live a double life in which they have to suppress the inner part of themselves or they stand up to their feelings and expose themselves to the conservative, popular outlook that society still has toward gay people. This generalized outlook reflects rejection and misunderstanding, often times even from family and friends.

Because of the loss of support from society, family and friends there is a natural need of finding other sources of self-recognition and love.

Multiple partners, and love making without love seems to be one source to overcome the pain they experience. Unfortunately they do not realize that the emotional part of their person is being raped.

Being openly gay in our society takes great courage. This courage will give those AIDS patients who are gay the inner-strength to heal themselves.

Drug users are also a "high risk" group for contracting AIDS. Drugs are an escape from reality, running away from oneself. This lifestyle effects the whole general strength of the body. They suffer from the deficiency of significant bonds and poor nutrition. Many drug users are searching for the once remembered and experience feeling of being one with the universe. They are usually very sensitive people.

But again, true healing can only be found within one's self. Self-acceptance and self-love will direct them to their path of contentment. Their sensitivity will help enable them to find their way back to themselves.

A high incidence of AIDS has also been seen in the Haitian population. A lack of self-recognition and self-love also exists amongst many of these people. They strive for identification within their society. Accepting and taking pride in their culture will help them to recognize their self-worth, and bring healing to their nation.

As our lifestyle deteriorates at a rapid pace, AIDS will express itself in the whole population.

Today, the fear of AIDS is as detrimental as AIDS itself. In an isolated case, 8 people tested positive for AIDS antibodies, 7 of them chose to take their own life. Fortunately, this is not an everyday occurance. The fact that it happened, is once to often.

The press, radio and TV, as well as the medical establishment are increasing the negative forces of fear throughout the whole population by suppressing positive information of healing, courage and love.

People, everyone, you and I, are searching for love. The love that we all need can only be found within. It is self-love. To turn within is to become peaceful and spiritual. To look without is to be materialistic. Money, possession and social esteem have no part of inner contentment. They are passing things and have no lasting value. Only within can everlasting happiness be found.

The self-love one usually has, can be destroyed easily by feelings of guilt and/or nonacceptance. Self-love means to love yourself as you are unconditionally. Do nice things for yourself. Start to love yourself today.

When one increases self-love, one can help and love his/her neighbor more by an increased understanding of each others differences. Peace can flourish in an environment of self-love. Those who bring love to the lives of others cannot keep it from themselves.

We are not speaking of vanity or narcissism. It is not an egotistical kind of love that we believe will make the difference, but a feeling of self-worth and the awareness of your created state of perfectability as a spiritual being, that will begin the dawn of a New Age.

AIDS is a dis-ease in which one has to go back to him/herself. We do not believe there will be a pill that relieves this malady. This time we will become our own healers.

AIDS will AID us to look within, then real healing can take place, and spiritual growth can occur.

AIDS is not only expressed in people. Mother Earth also has an "immune deficiency problem." After many years of abuse, she needs AID to heal herself from the wounds. Tuning into yourself with self-love, and appreciating Mother Earth will send her healing vibrations.

When AIDS is the recourse of bringing people back to themselves and their true destiny, then AIDS is **truly** a blessing and not a curse for our society.

Yes, there is hope! There are people who have healed themselves of AIDS by alternative methods of healing. If they can do it, so can you.

AIDS will AID us in bringing about change —where people will learn to love themselves, and express this love with healthy interactions between People, Mother Earth, and the Universe.

AIDS provides great hope and a chance for a spiritual revolution which will establish peace on earth!

AIDS is truly the miracle of the twentieth century!

HOW TO USE UROPATHY

There are several ways of approaching this therapy. It is extremely important to understand the benefits from internal as well as external usage. Let us first discuss the internal usage.

The amount of urine intake depends largely on the diseased state of the body and the will to recover.

People who start this treatment with the intent of ridding themselves of a malady, may fast on their urine. The longevity of the fast depends on the severity of one's health condition.

It is not believed long fasts are necessary to root our disease, but in certain cases it is strongly advocated to take short fast on urine and water, followed by a very light cleansing diet. This will considerably accelerate the speed of recovery time. **Anyone intending to fast should consult his/her physician before doing so.**

The method is quite simple. The only variation is the amount of urine intake, depending upon ones personal needs.

The amount of excreted urine, its concentration and taste

depend largely on diet and liquid intake. It also is related to the blood concentration and hormonal balance which in turn depend on diet and liquid intake.

The normal taste of urine will be salty and slightly bitter. Depending on food intake it may vary from very bitter and sour to almost sweet. Also the hormonal balance of a woman may influence the taste of urine — ex. just before menstruation it may taste more sour than normal.

The color of urine will also change. Normally, a completely healthy person's color of urine will range from clear, or colorless to an amber shade. The color variations from light to dark is indicative of the substances in the urine as well as liquid and diet intake the previous day. One can see with the human eye some of the cells and substances in the urine.

It is recommended to keep a diary with the daily intake of food and liquids as well as one with the taste of urine. Then compare the two lists and find the correlations between more unpleasant urine with certain foods. This way one can adjust his/her diet to their own specific needs. Urine not only supplies one with vital elements and essential substances, but will also increase the awareness of the quality of food one is eating. It will raise the conciousness of eating and drinking to the point where every meal will be a feast and celebration of life.

The first morning urine is the most efficacious against combating dis-ease and maintaining optimum health. The rationale is that after the body has rested during the night, the accumulation of minerals, hormones and vital elements contained in the urine are in higher concentration, making the first morning urine the most potent elixir.

One may observe this phenomenon by comparing the first morning urine to the ones passed throughout the day and evening. Usually the color becomes much lighter as the day progresses.

Upon rising in the morning, one should drink all his/her urine, excluding the beginning of the flow and end of the flow. The philosophy behind drinking the middle catch is that if there are any undesirable elements in the urine, they are excreted in the beginning and end of the flow. It is the cleanest and most sterile catch.

Healthy people may drink only their first morning urine daily and maintain optimum health. It should be noted that if there are any hidden maladies at the time of initiation, they will also be eradicated during the process of organic purification. One who is healthy may also experience some reactions as the body starts to cleanse itself.

Anyone else who is in a dis-eased state is strongly encouraged to take an increased dosage. All the urine one may pass daily or any increase in the amount will be more effective toward a speedy recovery. A note for those who are in need of intense healing from terminal dis-eases. These bodies are in need of a radical catharsis, drink all the urine passed, until the body reaches the point where it is eliminating a colorless urine.

If the urine is extremely dark and/or salty all day long, the recommendation would be to ingest all that is passed daily, stopping only when one rests during the night.

We would like to reiterate about one's diet. For purposes of healing a terminal dis-ease we strongly recommend that light, easily digestable foods be used in conjunction with this therapy. Plenty of fresh, pure water is also vital for healing purposes.

If one should find that during the course of the day he/she begins to urinate excessively, then the body has consumed enough for that day as long as its light amber to colorless. There is no need to overtax your kidneys by filtering more urine than necessary.

Intermittent use of urine is encouraged in the beginning to anyone who is not mentally comfortable with the therapy. Drinking it once or twice then going off it for a while has been done. Many times we have heard stories of external usage for long periods of time before actual ingestion took place. We have also heard stories of how one started UROPATHY and then abandoned it because they became frightened by some of the possible reactions, returning to it after their confidence and faith was restored. A tip for those of you who are finding it outrageously repulsive to make the initial ingestion, we have found that a chaser of pure water and brushing ones teeth after swallowing, eliminates any taste of urine from lingering in the mouth. After the first time one will find that it is like drinking warm salty water. Another thing to consider is how many times we have taken medications prescribed to us by medical doctors that have tasted obnoxious. The benefits derived from UROPATHY far exceed the salty or sour taste one experiences by drinking it.

A NOTE OF CAUTION:

Uropathy is strongly discouraged while on any kind of prescribed medications or recreational drugs. A combination of these drugs and UROPATHY may be hazardous to your health.

UROPATHY is to be used only in conjuction with herbs, vitamins, and other natural methods of healing, such as homeopathy, naturopathy, crystal healing etc.

EXTERNAL USAGE

The skin is the largest organ in the body. It is capable of excreting waste and sweat as well as absorbing fluids.

It is essential that one uses urine externally when using it internally. Urine's antiseptic qualities are unsurpassable.

The most important areas that urine should be rubbed or massaged on are the heart, head, neck, face, and feet. This does not mean however that other areas of the body should be neglected. Rubbing the entire body every morning with fresh urine will be a great asset for the skin. Nobody will smell your new lotion.

Urine is a skin-food and will rebuild tissues. It will also alleviate palpitations that might occur while fasting on it, in which case one should rub some on the chest area.

The skin will glow and become lustrous; the hair will become shiny. Wash the eyes with it; it has been known to strengthen the eyesight. Urine may be applied to bed sores, cuts, boils, wounds, lumps, swellings, or other abberations, as well as any skin dis-ease.

Soaking a cloth in urine, placing it over the affected area and remoistening it with urine when needed will provide for accelerated healing.

The use of old urine is suggested for wounds, rashes or any other skin lesions. Urine can be 3-4 days old, and stored at regular room temperature, so that fermentation can take place. Old urine has a very strong odor. It is suggested leaving it on for an hour then washing it off with mild soap and water.

Urine may also be used topically with herbal preparations, and poultices. The benefits of external usage of urine has been popular for centuries. In Europe, one of the old folk remedies was for a woman to apply a baby's diaper soaked with urine on her face, as well as rubbing it all over the infants body. This was reknown for radiant glowing complexions and exceptionally soft and supple skin.

REACTIONS TO UROPATHY

In this chapter we will discuss some of the possible reactions one may experience with UROPATHY.

Urine, when taken internally, will start to cleanse your body. This process is called "organic purification". The toxins must be eliminated.

Your body will begin to detoxify, purging all the toxins and poisonous matter, using every means possible in which to do so.

You may experience any of the following reactions:

- Vomitting or nausea
- Migraine headache
- Boils or pimples
- Skin rashes
- Palpitations
- Diarrhea
- A general feeling of uneasiness
- Fever

Any of these afformentioned reactions may occur. We cannot emphasize enough that one should not be frightened by these reactions. They are **NORMAL.**

The body must go through organic purification to reach optimum health. In order to do so, elimination of the toxic build-up must be expelled through the body's own natural mechanisms.

In all the case histories we have studied it is a mandatory step in the process of natural healing.

Everyone's chemical make-up is unique, therefore the rate and intensity at which purification and reactions occur will vary for each individual.

Some people go through this process quite quickly and easily, others will find it necessary to make radical changes in their diet and lifestyle. This will depend largely on how toxic one is.

There are basically three ways through which the body rids itself of toxins: skin, colon, and mouth.

1) Skin — The skin is one of the most important organs in the body for elimination. This may manifest itself in the form of rashes, sweating, fever, boils, pimples, and swelling —any way it can release toxins.

2) Colon — The elimination of toxins through the colon may occur with diarrhea. This can be a very strong diarrhea or a very easy flow of one feces. One may also experience some flatulence.

3) Mouth — Vomitting can occur or just simply the purge of fumes. One may also expel accumulated mucous from the lungs.

All these reactions may begin within a short time (2-3 days) or may take longer, depending upon one's health condition.

Some toxins may be expelled very quickly, other will take time to surface. It took several years for the body to become weak and vulnerable to dis-ease; have patience with the body's cleansing process. It is not uncommon for a recurrance of any of these reactions during the use of UROPATHY. In other words, even after the initial purge of toxins are eliminated, the body will continue to detoxify itself. If there are any residual or new toxins accumulating they will eventually be excreted. So, it is possible to have reactions even after six months or a year.

It' is recommended to continue the intake of urine during the time of reactions. In very extreme cases of diarrhea, a decreased intake of urine is indicated, making it easier for the body to adjust to this process. However, one should always use urine externally no matter what the amount of urine intake is.

The more dis-eased one is, the greater the reaction to the treatment, and a longer period of ingestion of urine will be needed to complete the healing process.

Even though the reactions seem to be incompatible in their appearance, think of what the body is doing at that time, and feel positive about it.

When the reactions appear to be too strong for one to handle, decrease the intake of urine; increase it again when one feels more at ease.

HERBS AND VITAMINS

In this chapter we would like to encourage the use of NATURALLY derived food supplements, namely herbs and vitamins, to enhance the quality of your lifestyle and promote healthy living.

First we will discuss Nature's miracle plants. Mother Earth provides for us many healing and nutritive plants, with medicinal qualities that far surpass modern drugs.

The great remedial properties of herbs have been recognized and appreciated since time began. It was not until the advent of the pharmaceutical companies that people have been diverted from the true healing remedies by superfluos advertising. False science has succeeded, as chemical poisons are quick-acting. People have been deceived for a long time. However, in this day, and for some time now, people are seeing the effects of drugs, and the evil after effects. They are looking for something better.

WHY USE HERBS? Herbal healing was the first system of healing that the world knew. They are nature's remedies and have been put here by an all-wise Creator. There is an herb for every dis-ease that the human body can be afflicted with. The use of herbs is the oldest medical science. Herbs were mentioned in the bible from the beginning of creation. Much has been written about herbs all through history.

There are literally thousands of herbs and this is not a book written merely about them, however, we will list a few of the most prominent herbs that can be used successfully in conjunction with UROPATHY.

For female troubles such as yeast infections, vaginitis, leucorrhea, and any internal vaginal problems, including herpes and venereal dis-ease, make a strong herbal solution of Golden Seal and urine. First, boil water as if making tea, shut off water and add 1/8 c. of Golden Seal powder. After this mixture has cooled, dilute it with enough water to make a little over a half gallon, then add enough urine to make a full gallon of solution. We found that an empty water jug works well and can be stored quite easily. Use this as a douche three times a day, or until symptoms disappear. Personal use of this method has proven successful. Golden Seal is one of the most wonderful and reknowned herbs. It excels in its effectiveness against a host of other ailments including stomach and liver trouble, skin dis-ease, and inflamations. It exerts a special influence on all mucous membranes and tissues with which it comes in contact. Combined with Scullcap and Red Pepper (Cayenne) it will greatly relieve and strengthen the heart. It also has no superior when combined with Myrrh, one part Golden Seal, to one-fourth Myrrh for ulcerated stomach, and duodenum. It is especially good for enlarged tonsils and sores in the mouth. It has also been known to be used in cases of skin cancer with excellent results. As one can see, the list of uses for this herb is very extensive, and considering all that can be accomplished by its use, it does seem like a real cure-all.

A combination of Ginger and urine, when taken hot, can be extremely useful for supressed menstruation, eradicating colds and flu, chronic bronchitis, and excessive mucous in the lungs. We usually boil water then add Ginger as if making tea (use less when using fresh Ginger Root) and add a small amount of urine (about 2 oz.) after the water has boiled. Let stand for a few minutes to cool off, then drink as you would a glass of tea. This mixture of Ginger and urine has been proven to be extremely effective for sore throats, fever, and symptoms associated with cold and flu season, as well as sinus problems.

Short fasts on urine and Ginger are often recommended to promote a speedy recovery from colds and flu, as well as a general detoxifier.

With more pressure at home and on the job, many people have increased stress levels existent in their lives today. Now, more than ever, doctors are prescribing tranquilizers and drugs to their patients to help them cope with the stress of their daily lives. Insomnia, nervous tension, headaches, lack of vitality, poor digestion, and extreme fatigue are just a few of the symptoms associated with the socioeconomic pressures of today's society. Many people are dissatisfied with their working environment. This has had a profound effect on their health.

Valium and librium are two of the most widely prescribed tranquilizers on the market today. The side effects from these drugs can be most dangerous, not to mention the thousands of people addicted to them.

After studying herbology for many years, the most fascinating thing to discover was that many of these synthetic drugs were derived from natural sources. Why not leave nature alone?!

Valium is derived from an herb called Valerian Root, which when taken in its unaltered state produces the same sedative effects as valium, without the addictive properties or harmful side effects. Many of our patients and clients have switched over to Valerian finding the results more optimal. They not only sleep better, but enjoy waking up in the morning without that heavy head feeling one incurs by taking valium. When Valerian is mixed with Scullcap, Lady's Slipper, Chamomile, Hops, and other nervines it promotes peaceful sleep and relaxes the nerves. There are many commercially prepared nervine tonics containing these combinations in your local health food store. Experience for yourself the benefits of Mother Nature's own pharmacy.

For acute cases of insomnia and palpitations of the heart, rubbing urine on the chest and abdomen before bed, together with the use of these herbs has been highly acclaimed and experienced personally.

For dis-eases of the skin like Poison ivy, rashes, eczema, psoriasis, pimples, acne, boils, warts, skin-cancer, and any others not mentioned here, the best and most effective herbs known are Comfrey and Aloe. Nature's healing process is usually slower, but longer lasting, and less dangerous. When one combines urine with these two herbs it accelerates the healing of skin disorders at a rapid pace. Cases of poison ivy and sun poisoning were taken away within a couple of days after topical application of a mixture of these herbs and urine.

One last herb we felt would be advantageous to your health is Stinging Nettle. It is reknown for relief of edema, swelling, water retention, and it purifies the blood and kidneys. We found that short fasts on urine and Stinging Nettle increases the flow of urine; it acts as a diuretic.

As one can see, there are many uses for herbs. They can be taken and obtained quite easily. Give nature a chance! One thing to remember when using herbal preparations is to use them with prudence and thanksgiving. After all they are a gift from Mother Earth and our Creator. Allow time for healing. One cannot rush the natural process of healing. Recite some positive affirmations and meditate while using herbs; healing will take place.

We further encourage you to educate yourselves in the wonderful field of herbology. You will be truly amazed at the documented success stories. Books on this topic can be found in the back of this book under Suggested Resources.

Important reminder: *Never use aluminum pots to prepare your herbal remedies.*

The next topic to discuss in this chapter is vitamins. Vitamins have become a multi-billion dollar industry. With the media hype and thousands of publicized books, articles, and health professionals advocating the use of them, it is easy to see why sales have reached these proportions.

Vitamins can be very beneficial to one's health if used properly. Ideally, all our vitamins, minerals, and other nutrients should be obtained from the foods we eat. Since we know this is not possible, due to the toxification of our foods through the use of insecticides, chemicals, and now the process of irradiation, we must take extra precautionary measures to insure proper consumption of vital elements. The nutritionally inferior and poisonous foods of today cause many nutritional deficiencies, derangement of body chemistry, and lower resistance to dis-ease.

The prime purpose of food supplements is to fill the nutritional gaps produced by faulty eating habits and by nutritionally inferior foods. The therapeutic value of vitamins in the treatment of dis-ease also has much merit and can be of tremendous help in fighting dis-ease and accelerate speedy recovery.

The first thing we must do is make a distinction between natural and synthetic vitamins. Most drug-store quality vitamins are made from synthetic chemicals — they are not derivatives of natural food substances. Although this is also true of some brands sold in health food stores, most brands sold in health food stores are concentrations of nutrients from such natural sources as rose hips, green peppers, acerola berries (vitamin C); brewers yeast, liver, or rice polishings (vitamin B); fish liver oil, or lemon grass (vitamin A and D); vegetable oils (vitamin E); kelp (iodine); bone meal, egg shells and milk (minerals); etc.

There is a great deal of controversy regarding the difference and usefullness of synthetic vs. natural vitamins. Natural health authorities usually claim that synthetic vitamins are useless, ineffective, and even harmful. Most orthodox doctors and dieticians claim that synthetic vitamins have a molecular structure identical to the so-called natural vitamins, and that they are just as effective. Who is right?

An intelligent solution to the problem seems to be as follows: On the whole we can trust nature further than the chemist and his synthetic vitamins. We must keep in mind that in nature vitamins are never isolated. They are always present in the form of vitamin complexes. When you take natural vitamins, you are getting all the vitamins and vitamin-like factors that naturally occur in these foods —that is all those that are already discovered as well as those that are not yet discovered.

Our knowledge of vitamins is not complete. New vitamins are discovered frequently. When you take vitamins in the form of vitamin-rich supplements, or in the form of "complexes", you are getting the benefit of all the known as well as unknown vitamins.

For those who are confused as to which vitamins are synthetic and which are natural we advise reading the labels. As a general rule, if the formula on the bottle does not say that the vitamin is natural or is derived from natural source, it is synthetic. Companies list fancy chemical names to confuse the customer from making an intelligent choice. The FDA (Food and Drug Administration) allows anything containing 5% natural and 95% synthetic ingredients to be called 100% natural. You must be an expert label reader even in a health food store!

Another factor to take into consideration when purchasing food supplements is that the vitamins are in an easily assimilable form. Many scientific studies reveal that a large percentage of vitamins are excreted in the urine. These vitamins when recycled by drinking one's own urine can be very economical. A very minute amount is actually assimilated and absorbed by the body. This is one of the reasons why people find it necessary to ingest mega-doses of vitamins to exhibit noticeable results. We do not advocate taking mega-doses of vitamins, but what we do support is buying vitamins in chelated, liquid orotate, or powder form, so they can be assimilated much quicker, and therefore are more beneficial for utilization in your body.

Taking vitamin and mineral supplements seems to be a necessary measure in proper health care in today's society. They should be integrated into one's daily life, especially if the diet consists of the popular, typical American junk and fast food diet.

UROPATHY works well when taking vitamin supplements. As we mentioned before it can be very cost effective. You can recycle all the vitamins contained in your urine. We know several people who do, and they have found the need to decrease their intake of vitamins because of feeling well nourished and balanced.

You can become familiar with each vitamin and the reasons why particular vitamins are indicated to combat certain dis-eases. It is part of the complete holistic approach to healing. Top educational material about vitamins are listed in Suggested Resources.

HEALTHY LIFESTYLE

The human body is an amazing organism. The innate wisdom of the body knows exactly how to digest food and make living cells out of the nutrients. Everytime you eat, the perfect amount of stomach acid is produced. The different enzymes are responsible for putting the right nutrients into the right places. Your heart is pumping blood through your system to nourish and oxygenate every part of your body. We even produce our own elixir for optimum health.

All these reactions occur automatically without thinking about it. Actually the less intervention the body has, the better it works.

Our responsibility is to take care of this fantastic vehicle called the body. Unfortunately, one goes through many years of formal education, but never really learns the most obvious and important task —to take care of one's own body.

In the 1980's, this is not an easy and simple task. Today one has to learn the tricks of the trade to understand the labels on our food packages. Keep informed of what the government is doing, otherwise your freedom will be less by the year! Examples of decreasing freedom are required immunization for school children, which has detrimental effects for many, the outlaw of raw milk sales, limiting successful holistic health care providers by revoking their licenses, and irradiating foods etc. Today one has to stand up for his/her rights. Standing united we are strong. Together we keep freedom of choice in health care and food supplies. The National Health Federation, the largest such organization in America, lobbies for these rights.

Let us take a look at what proper health care should include:

1) A healthy naturally-derived diet
2) Plenty of fresh air and water
3) Moderate exercise (any form)
4) Personal natural hygiene
5) Meditation or prayer

Everything you put in and on your body will have some effect on the way it functions and performs.

The human body was not designed to digest and absorb many of the harmful additives we are exposed to everyday. Chemicals and radiation added to the foods we eat have demonstrated further abuse to our bodies.

A suggested diet would contain fresh vegetables, fresh fruits, whole grains, seeds, nuts, beans, natural sweetners, such as honey, and a limited intake of dairy products.

Not recommended is anything made of white flour, white rice, and white sugar. Excessive consumption of meat and white sugar is directly connected with high levels of cholesterol and heart dis-ease. Try substituting fish and fowl that has not been given hormones. Avoid anything processed, irradiated, artificially colored and/or flavored. Your diet should be as individual as you are. Experiment and see what type of diet fits your lifestyle while giving you the highest energy level possible.

It is almost impossible to totally escape the poisons that permeate our existence. We must take extra precautionary measures to insure our health.

Fresh air and water are vital to a person's health. Getting good, healthy water is not that easy anymore. Usually the tap water contains fluoride, chloride and aluminum, to mention only a few. Bottled water is strongly recommended for drinking and cooking purposes.

Our lakes and oceans become more and more polluted by the waste products from our lifestyle. Water is an essential living substance. If we do not take care of it now, it will not take care of us later!

The same holds true for our air. The sky is not a dump for poisonous gases. Air is essential for breathing and living.

Heavy traffic areas like big cities are not a place to do jogging and breathing excercises. An ideal place for healthy air is a wooded area.

Yes, fresh air and pure water are rare commodities these days, but it is possible to obtain both, if they lie high on your list of priorities. Health is the most important asset in life. INSURING YOUR HEALTH IS YOUR RESPONSIBILITY. It seems that many people have lost their health while striving to obtain material possessions. Health is wealth!

Exercise includes any movement of the body that speeds up the heart rate, promotes circulation, and increases muscle tone. There are innumerable ways to achieve this goal. What is important is that it becomes part of your daily routine. Make exercising a fun part of your life. Even if you choose to do something different everyday, you will benefit from any type of increased movement.

Personal natural hygiene is something that everyone must be more conscious of.

The mass manufactured products that people use to clean their bodies contain many harmful chemicals and ingredients. It almost appears to be intentional when you have doctors representing these products which will in turn cause you ill-health. Something really astounding is the way dentists will advocate the use of toothpaste, which has sugar as one of the ingredients. What a hoax!

Your shampoos, deodorants, soaps, toothpastes, and body lotions, not to mention the cosmetics that woman apply on their skin daily, are all laden with toxic chemicals.

It makes common sense that if you spray your underarms daily with the commercial brand deodorants you are spraying directly into your lymph nodes cancer-causing chemicals. They are absorbed through the skin. What about all the body lotions with artificial colors? These lotions are also absorbed through the skin. The products that you clean your body with should be natural and nourishing to your body. They will seep through the skin and ultimately have to be assimilated in some form. Your colon and other vulnerable areas are where these toxins build up in your body. There must be some connection between this and dis-ease.

Just because a product is labeled "natural" does not mean that it is. Start reading the fine printed labels. You will be astonished at what the government (FDA) will allow products and foods to contain. In a health food store, one will find a plethora of body care products that contain natural ingredients and are just as effective, if not more so, in maintaining natural hygiene.

Mental hygiene is just as important as physical hygiene. The same way we clean our bodies or our houses, we should clean our thoughts. This starts with controlling the thoughts in our minds. Our thoughts are very powerful; thoughts play a large part in creating our reality. They can create happiness or sadness.

When one sees a glass half-filled with water, one can look at it either as half-empty or half-filled. When one is very thirsty a half-empty glass will be very depressive and negative, while a half-filled glass will make one more appreciative and positive. The amount of water stays the same.

There is no such thing as a bad day or a rainy, ugly day. The way we perceive it makes it good or bad, the day itself is neutral.

We are in control of our own thoughts and feelings, and we determine how we like to look at things.

We are very selective with the food we eat. It has to be fresh, pure, natural, and delicious. Thoughts are food for our inner-self. We should be just as selective with our thoughts. Only the pure, positive, peaceful and loving thoughts are good foods for your inner-self.

One way to learn to control and choose our thoughts is meditation. The more one exercises to create positive thoughts, the easier it will get, until it is a natural part of one's life.

Meditation is an art that must be developed. For some it may come quite naturally, others will need more discipline.

If you are not in the habit of or have never meditated before, here are a few tips that may help you. There are many ways in which to achieve results, find one that is compatible with your nature.

One must realize that prayer and meditation are very similar. The major difference is that prayer is done on a more conscious level and meditation is done on a subconscious level. The ultimate goal is not an appearance of God in a physical sense, but an interaction between the conscious mind and the higher realm.

As you develop your skills and awareness of the spiritual world, you find that the union of the physical and spiritual plane will open your eyes to a completely different perspective about life.

The first step one must take to meditate is to find a relaxing position for the physical body, so that one may lose all sense of it. The traditional lotus position, lying down, sitting, or even while taking a bath are helpful techniques. The important thing to accomplish when meditating is leaving your physical body behind as you connect your spirit with a higher energy.

The second step is to completely relax the body, letting the weight of the body sink with gravity. Take a few deep breaths, (inhale through the nose, exhale through the mouth) letting your stomach rise when you inhale, and deflate when you exhale.

The next thing to do is to let all thoughts, whatever they may be, run through your mind at random. Do not try and focus on one particular thought in the beginning. Letting these thoughts run through the mind as they come through, the impulses in the brain will have a calming effect on the body. As you become less aware of your breathing and your physical body, your mind will start to slow down. The whole process of thinking seems to stop. At this time it is helpful to focus on the third eye, or spiritual eye, located in the center of the forehead between the eyes. Try to concentrate on a beam of illuminous white light filling your whole body.

You will begin to focus on a few visions. Sometimes one vision or thought will become very strong and the mind will elaborate on it. You may also find yourself with no thoughts at all. Do not push yourself in either direction. Let the thoughts flow at will.

To be still and quiet in your mind is difficult to achieve at first, do not be discouraged. It will come to you with practice and discipline. At first you may be very easily distracted by little annoyances which keep you in your physical body. Conquering the awareness of your physical body is a giant step forward to a more uplifting meditation.

The calmer and quieter your mind becomes, the easier it is to make contact with the spiritual world. When you drink the water of life, it will enhance your meditations, and will channel your knowledge of the spiritual world at a rapid pace.

It is the union of the subconscious and conscious mind that can direct you on a lighted, uplifting path toward perfection and godliness.

Work on these steps and do not place heavy expectation on the meditation or yourself. No meditation is a failure. Each one is vitally important to your body's healing, balancing, and path of unfolded spiritual enlightenment.

Your meditations are unique and personal unto yourself. Be pleased and thankful with every little experience and progression. You will open yourself up quickly and easily with a positive attitude.

We believe that meditation is an integral part of healing the physical body. Be still and LISTEN!

In the back of this book we have included a list of suggested tapes and books which will further educate you in this area.

HOLISTIC HEALING

Starting on UROPATHY is the first step. Saying yes to yourself and to self-love initiates the process of healing. Healing must take place on three levels, the spiritual level, the physical level, and the emotional level.

1) Spiritual healing occurs when we become aware of our place and purpose in the universe. Dis-ease will manifest its way into our lives when we need to become re-aligned with the spirit and the will within, to become ONE with our creator. Believe in the power of the God energy and you will find it exists **within** your vehicle.

Many holy scriptures and literature, the yogis and the great spiritual masters of our time, tell us to look within for the answers to the mysteries of the universe. We are the universe! We are the miracle! Anytime we are in need of healing, the spiritual aspect is part of the complete holistic approach, and must be integrated into one's life!

2) Physical Healing encompasses exercise, sunshine, fresh air, and any activity of the physical body at a moderate level depending upon your state of health and the amount of physical activity you are presently doing. You need not be an olympic athlete. Walking, jogging, swimming, biking —there are literally thousands of ways to exercise. Nevertheless, it must be a part of your routine whatever you choose, otherwise atrophy of the muscles and decreased vitality will result.

The other area of physical healing that needs to be addressed is nutrition. We believe it is necessary to reemphasize a recommended diet since it plays such a major role in the body's healing powers. We advocate a natural food diet. This excludes any type of processed food, artificially colored or flavored food, and denatured food of any kind. Chemicals, preservatives, white sugar, white flour, white rice, heavy consumption of meats and salty foods should be avoided. The body was not designed to assimilate these foreign substances. They accumulate in your colon and cause a toxic build-up. This will be the onset of a myriad of dis-eases.

At the same time we do not advocate any type of extreme diet unless you have already made the transition and feel comfortable with your eating habits. Sometimes making a transition from eating unhealthy foods to a healthy diet overnight may be a shock to the system and inflict a radical catharsis. A slow process of elimination is recommended, until you become familiar with healthy substitutes to insure proper and adequate consumption of the essential minerals, vitamins and amino acids of a balanced, healthy diet.

Foods we recommend are fresh fruits and fresh vegetables (steamed or raw), whole grains, seeds, nuts, beans, cold pressed oils, soybean products, fish, untainted fowl, and any of the following natural sweetners which can be substituted for white sugar: maple syrup, honey, barley malt, rice syrup, molasses, fructose, and fruit juices.

A note for those of you who are lactose intolerant; you will find a large selection of cheeses, yogurts, milk, and other dairy substitutes made from soy products, that are extremely delicious, in your local health food store.

Experiment by shopping in health food stores. You will be surprised at what you find, and you will have fun doing it. It may seem more expensive at first, but after you eliminate some meat from your diet you will see the cost is essentially the same or less.

3) Emotional healing will be the evolution of the mind. We have been inundated with many schools of thought, theories, customs and cultures, depending upon our background. From the day we are born we are taught our parents ideals. We are conditioned over centuries to believe that the body excretes filth and waste. We have lost the true meaning behind our very existence —perfection! The healing powers lie within us. We are only as powerful and as perfect as we allow ourselves to think we are. The imagination has no boundaries; it is limitless. We can do anything that our imagination perceives.

Meditation and relaxation are excellent ways to promote the process of emotional healing. Recommended tapes and books are listed in suggested resources to further your awareness of the power of the imagination and to assist your spiritual growth and inner development.

We must break through these mental barriers and recondition our thought patterns back to the time when nature ruled the planet.

It is our responsibility to see that harmony is restored in Us, Mother Earth, and the Universe.

UROPATHY is the key to healing of the body, mind and spirit.

OUR SELF-INVOLVEMENT

Dr. Beatrice Bartnett

As a Naturopathic and Chiropractic Physician, I am quite open to any method of healing which show results. I believe very strongly in the innate wisdom of the body and appreciate all the healing substances Mother Earth provides us with.

It was for reason that I was exposed to this unusual therapy. I saw miracles happen. A strong urge pushed me to do more research.

After finding scientific back-up on the theory of URO-PATHY, I was compelled to do further case-studies. With what I know I cannot close my eyes and fit into my beloved profession anymore for "truth" shall be revealed in our time.

It was not easy to expose myself involved with something totally different and unusual. I know that I will get oppositon from very strong associations. The more people that become knowledgeable and experience this gift, the stronger it will stay alive.

Exposing you to this truth helps me to share with you the responsibility we all have for mankind.

UROPATHY is not just drinking the Water of Life, but further more a lifestyle, which will enhance you spiritually, emotionally and physically. I would like to thank everyone who sent me positive vibrations to give me the courage to stand up for this great gift and my beliefs.

Margie Adelman, L.M.T., C.N.

I have been drinking my own urine daily for the past four years. I do not believe in coincidences or accidents. I believe I was guided by a higher energy source to discover a most remarkable, fascinating and indisputable truth. There are many universal truths. I believe urine with its miraculous healing powers, is one of them. In my opinion this is the link between science and religion.

It all started when I was working at a health food restaurant in Miami. A woman whom I had always admired for her mystical nature saw me with a cold sore on my lip. She said, "If you apply some urine it will heal right up." At first I was a little skeptical, but I decided to take her advice, and it worked! The cold sore had vanished within two days of applying the urine. That was the last I heard of UROPATHY for two years.

My life took me on a path to Los Angeles, California. While living in L.A. I became acutely hypoglycemic. At that time, my only knowledgeable means of controlling low blood sugar was through my diet. I continued this treatment until I was exposed to UROPATHY again at a later date.

Returning to Florida, two years later, I met another person who had a profound effect on my life. In search of a career in the health field, I came across an ad for reflexology courses. I set out to inquire about the classes. When I arrived at the address, I found a little house, with animals running about, and an elderly man. Nervous, I quickly asked the man about the reflexology classes. He told me he held classes on Sundays, but that he was not state certified. I explained to him that I was looking for more professional type training, an accredited school, so I could become licensed. In the midst of our conversation, and without hesitation, this eccentric old man looked me in the eye and said, "you ought to be drinking your own urine. I have been taking in my waters daily for over three years." He gave me a book called the "Water of Life" by J.W. Armstrong. I proceeded to read the book in record time. The very next day, I started using my urine externally for about two months.

I remembered the woman in the health food restaurant. I decided to ask her if she had ever heard of consuming one's own urine. When I confronted her with it, she said, "Oh, yes, I have been drinking my waters every day for over six years."

That was enough for me, somehow it all seemed so logical. I immediately began drinking my own urine. The first two weeks I experienced a moderate amount of diarrhea, a little nausea, and a few headaches. These reactions were just a natural response to the body's detoxification. I had already experienced similar symptoms from previous times when I had fasted. By about the 3rd or 4th week I felt much better and all discomforts had subsided.

My friend and I spoke often, and the more we talked, the more I believed in what I was doing. She lent me a book on urine therapy called "Shivambu Kalpa." Reading this book, which is now completely out of print, I became even more confident and positive. Since then, I have been drinking my urine everyday with occasional short terms fasts.

I have only told a handful of people about this therapy since I started because of its controversial and anti-social nature. I did, however, speak frequently with my friend at the health food restaurant and returned back to the elderly man, in search for more evidence supporting UROPATHY.

About a year later, the elderly man disclosed a book to me that is without a doubt the most powerful and truthful book I have ever layed my hands on. Thanks to my persistence, several months later I received my own copy. The book is entitled, "The Lost Gospel of the Ages, Key to Immortality and Companion to the Holy Bible."

This book was compiled by a man whom I have yet to meet despite futile attempts. His name is John Christian Androgeous. I would like to personally thank him for keeping the truth alive, through his courageous work. Your persistence has finally paid off. Congratulations!

This book is a compilation of ancient scripts and literature written by secret orders and religious organizations that used urine therapy amongst their people. The evidence is overwhelming and astounding. It also contains literature like the Dead Sea Scrolls, Alchemical Texts of the Hermetic Brothers, the Gospel of Christian Alchemy, the Keys of Free Masonry and many other writings that can be interpreted or connected with the use of urine as a sacred elixir. This book is truly a learning tool to re-educate humanity about philosophy, religion, man, and the universe.

I believe that people should study this book intensively to find out the deception this world has been under for a long period of time. True interpretation of the Bible has been hidden for centuries. Misconceived perceptions about symbology is the basis for our misunderstanding, confusion, and blind faith that pervades society today.

I believe it is my mission to unveil this knowledge, and my responsibility to do so.

The story of how Dr. Bartnett and I met is a prime example of destiny, fate, and karma.

One of my friends, who lives in New York, had asked me to come and speak to a group of people concerning UROPATHY. I was quite hesitant at first, but he was relentless, and finally persuaded me to do it. He had scheduled me to speak almost a month in advance. When I went to the travel agency to pick up my ticket, they had no record of my reservation. The earliest flight available would put me in to New York 3 hours too late. The only thing to do was to call my friend and tell him I could not make it. When I contacted him and told him my dilemma, he told me to come anyhow.

I arrived at his house in New York after a delayed flight about 1:00 A.M. When I got there I was totally exhausted. My friend pointed out Dr. Bartnett to me and said that she had been doing some work in Switzerland with URO-

PATHY. She had come to listen to my lecture but ended up giving it. There were still some people waiting there to hear my personal experience with UROPATHY, so I proceeded to talk.

After I finished, Dr. Bartnett told me I did a great job. We revealed to each other that we were both presently writing a book on this subject. We decided to collaborate. The amazing thing was that she had obtained scientific evidence, while I had obtained a metaphysical back-up. We complimented each other in so many ways. Our strongest bond was that we both had seen the miracles of UROPATHY.

It was at this time that Dr. Bartnett and I began giving seminars and working with AIDS patients using UROPATHY.

This story may seem quite coincidental to some, but when it happens to you, you know that it is not! We found our encounter quite amazing. There were forces which brought Dr. Bartnett and me together to produce this book which may revolutionize the method of healing in this country, and hopefully all over the world.

CASE HISTORY AND TESTIMONIALS

Margie's Self-Cure

Earlier in the book, I mentioned that I had hypoglycemia. It was not long after I started UROPATHY that I noticed my symptoms fading away one by one. Before I started, I could not go for long periods of time without eating food. My blood sugar was very unstable, and at that point my diet was extremely disciplined. I could not understand why my body was not totally healed. Occassionally I would feel extremely enervated, and had palpitations, profuse sweating, and shortness of breath. These are all common symptoms of hypoglycemia. I had been to doctors and was thoroughly disgusted with the treatment they prescribed. At one point I remember trying a prescribed diet by a renown doctor in California, who was suppose to be nutritionally oriented. I never felt worse! After one week on this diet I was constipated and felt totally disoriented, and unbalanced. So, I set out to heal myself, and found a very compatible diet to my vegetarian eating habits. The book, "Hypoglycemia, A Better Approach" by Paavo Airola saved my life. But even after nine months of strict eating, I still felt that the hypoglycemia was not totally eradicated.

After only two months on UROPATHY, I began to feel normal again. I was able to go off my diet and not feel the consequences afterward. Slowly but surely I was getting better. To this day, four years later, I haven't had any problems with my blood sugar level, and I feel more energetic and robust than I did when I was 20 years old.

Another phenomenon that occurred was that my skin cleared up. I never had acne problems, but had occasional breakouts that disturbed me. When I began applying urine to may face and skin I noticed that my skin got extremely smooth, my hair got shinier, and my complexion was glowing and radiant like never before. I am also able to fast a few days on urine and watermelon juice; before I started UROPATHY it was totally out of the question. My blood sugar level fell so quickly that I knew I had to eat or I was going to pass out.

Thanks to UROPATHY I am able to continue a healthy lifestyle, whereas before, I really believe I was headed for some serious medical problems.

COLLECTED DATA

Miss D. of Florida

This woman has juvenile diabetes. After ingesting her urine for about a month, she has found she can eliminate her evening dose of insulin. She tested her blood sugar constantly. About a month later has reported that she is ready to even further reduce her insulin intake. While she was using urine externally as well, she noticed her varicose veins starting to diminish. After two weeks of frequent topical applications, there is only a trace left. She is feeling very well, and has had no other problems while on UROPATHY.

Mr. J. of Florida

This man has had fungal growth on his foot for over a year. After just 3 days of rubbing urine on his foot, he reports that he cannot believe how fast it healed. He has tried many of the creams and antibiotics, and none of them worked as quickly and as thoroughly as UROPATHY. He also cut his finger very deeply while working, and says that his finger healed within 48 hours. He used only urine therapy.

Mrs. D. of Florida

Very discouraged and completely dissatisfied with conventional medical treatment, this woman was seeking relief from sebaceous cysts. They were all over her face and neck. She had the cysts for over a year and had been to many doctors, taken medication, and applied countless creams on her skin. Totally fed up. she decided to try UROPATHY. After approximately one week, the cysts were opening and draining. She was so enthused that she kept up the daily rubbings and increased to three or four applications a day. All she did was rub urine over the cysts. She was amazed and delighted with her success. Almost all of the cysts were draining and she was forming new skin underneath. This happened over a three week time span. She continues to apply urine to her face and says her complexion never looked so good. We have noticed a definite positive change in her attitude toward life as well.

Miss A. from New York

Using UROPATHY internally for 3 months, once daily in the morning, she reports a clearer complexion and relief of poison ivy. She had no medical problems when she started UROPATHY. She noticed that she became aware of foods that agree and disagree with her.

Miss K. from New York

She has been using UROPATHY internally and externally for 3 month. She noticed weight loss, and improved skin condition. She also says that her diet has improved tremendously and attributes this to UROPATHY.

Mr. Q. from New York

He has been using UROPATHY internally and externally a little over 3 months. He had ringworm and athletes foot. He claims a sore throat as a reaction to UROPATHY, but it subsided very quickly. He also reveals that he cured his athletes foot, has had relief of mouth ulcers and dissolved a ganglion cyst in his wrist. He says he feels stronger and healthier.

Mr. N. from New York

Has been using UROPATHY for 2 1/2 weeks both internally and externally. He complained of chest, lung and sinus congestion. He now says that thanks to UROPATHY his lung congestion is gone, and his breathing is much easier.

Ms. D.A. from New York

Diagnosed with ARC. Has been using UROPATHY internally and externally for 2 months. She had the following reactions to UROPATHY: diarrhea, vomiting, rashes, and headaches. All reactions have subsided, and she feels she has a higher energy level. She was also diagnosed with hepatitis and recently her liver tests came back normal. We are still collecting data on this person.

Ms. J. from Connecticut

Has been using UROPATHY internally for 2 weeks. She reports that her circulation has increased and has better color in her cheeks.

Mr. C. from New York

Has been on UROPATHY for 4 months. Before he started he had athletes foot, perspiration, acne on back, and upset stomach. He experienced a sore throat and headache as a reaction to UROPATHY. He writes that he has a healthier body, better eating habits, glowing skin, and better muscle tone. He also states that all previously mentioned conditions have improved considerably.

Mr. R. from California

Has been using UROPATHY internally and externally for 1 month. He had the following health problems before starting: bloated stomach, gas, itchy rash, fatigue, susceptible to frequent colds, bumps on his head, and red blotches on his face, arms and legs. His reaction to UROPATHY was diarrhea and a skin rash of small red sores with white heads (pus). He says that all the reactions to UROPATHY have subsided and all the bloatedness and gas in stomach are gone, rash immediately started to disappear and bumps on his head disappeared rapidly. Furthermore he writes, that urine therapy came into his life to give him a chance to detoxify his body preparing himself for his spirit guide.

Mr. L. from New York

Diagnosed with Kaposi's Sarcoma, Cellulitis, and Edema. He has been using UROPATHY daily for 3 months internally and externally. He reports that he did not experience any related reactions to UROPATHY and attributes this to 10 consecutive weeks of high enemas (once weekly). Since he's been on UROPATHY the water retention in his thighs has been dismissed, the major modular lesions on left leg have come to a head, and opened, smaller lesion areas are experiencing rejuvination of the skin through a black and blueing process for 2 months. He finds that sustaining a healthy diet while on UROPATHY is keeping his cancer in a prolonged state of remission. He is now fasting on urine and utilizing external applications of urine for prolonged periods of time (1 1/2 to 2 hours). We are waiting to obtain further results from the fast he is presently undergoing.

Mrs. N. from Connecticut

Has been using UROPATHY internally and externally for three months. Detoxification mostly through the skin. Her energy level has increased drastically; her skin looks healthy and shiny. Her eyes are clear and she feels especially healthy after a urine and water fast, in which she does not experience any of the usual symptoms of a fast. On the contrary, she has more energy during a fast and does not feel hungry or weak.

Mrs. E. from Switzerland

Diagnosed with metastatic cancer of the liver, complicated by hepatitis. She was sent home to die. Mrs. E. started UROPATHY at home after the medical profession gave up any hope of recovery. She drank only her first morning urine and used it externally, no fasting. After 10 days she went back to the doctor; he could not believe she was still alive, and felt much better. Within a few weeks she was working again.

Mrs. B. from Switzerland

Diagnosed with an inoperable uterine tumor. She has been drinking all the urine she passed daily, and uses it externally. The tumor dissolved itself within 7 days; she was extremely excited about it.

Mr. R. from New York

Cut on his foot left him with several stitches, pain redness and swelling. By using urine externally every two hours the pain and redness disappeared and the swelling went down. After going back to the doctor, the patient got scared and was prescribed salve by the doctor, which again gave him pain, redness and swelling. Many people are intimidated by their doctors. Often it is difficult for the patients to decide to trust their own inner-wisdom.

Mrs. N. from Connecticut

She has very dry skin to the extent that she gets deep cracks. They are very painful and do not heal easily. External use of UROPATHY every two hours relieved the pain almost instantly and the cracks healed within 12 hours.

Ms. J. from Florida

She has been using UROPATHY for one month internally and externally. Before starting, she had an extremely bad case of varicose veins. After 2 weeks of external application the varicose veins started to disappear.

Mr. M. from New York

He has been using UROPATHY for 4 months internally and externally. He had poor digestion and mucous filled eyes before starting the therapy. He had diarrhea, boils and a cough as reactions to UROPATHY. After applying urine directly into his eyes for 3 days with an eye dropper his eyes are much clearer and brighter. There is no mucouses. Also believes that his muscle tone has improved immensely due to topical application. He also reports that his channeling has been enhanced greatly by UROPATHY and has opened him up more spiritually in many ways.

PERSONAL TESTIMONY ON THE EFFECTIVENESS OF URINE THERAPY

I am a recently diagnosed PWA (Person with AIDS) due to a biopsy confirmation in March of 1987 for one oral Kaposi's Sarcoma lesion.

For over 6 months I had been experiencing a virulent case of ringworm or athlete's foot (to this day undetermined), apparently resistant to standard anti-fungal creams, powders, etc.

During the course of each monthly doctor's appointment, I frustratingly shared with my doctor the fact that all medications applied directly to the foot were unsuccessful.

Toward the end of May, I had heard of a gathering taking place on "Urine Therapy for PWA's" and felt compelled to investigate. That's when I met Dr. Beatrice Bartnett (Switzerland) and her partner Margie Adelman (Florida), and had decided to investigate some of the anecdotes they were sharing.

I was of course immediately repulsed at the idea of drinking my own urine. My attention drifted as I closed my mind off from the rest of the discourse. Later, however, when Margie Adelman related her account of totally bringing a severe vaginal yeast infection under control simply by douching with her own urine, the wheels in my mind started turning. And as I listened attentively my hopes of having a viable alternative were reinforced by the numerous success stories that were shared with the audience. They ranged from eradication of a terminal cancer diagnosis to dissolving cysts and skin lesions associated with a whole slew of dis-eases and infections.

It was at this time that I raised my hand and asked if I could get relief from my own disturbing affliction by applying my urine directly to the foot. I was assured that I would almost immediately notice an improvement. Frankly, I could not wait to go home and begin.

That evening, before retiring, I applied my urine with a plantspray bottle. Later that evening, I noticed for the first time in months that my infected foot had not itched me into a frenzy. I would never scratch the site, but I always felt the tingling and itchy feeling all night long. That feeling was definitely absent!

For the next 2 days, I sprayed my right foot before putting on my work socks and shoes, almost creating a light urine compress at the bottom of my feet. Each evening I noticed that not only was there no longer any sensitivity or itching, but that the infection site was disappearing completely.

At the base of my toes on the underside of the foot, I also had a terrible case of breaking, cracked skin, as if psoriasis. The urine had also cleared this up, to the point that even the texture and color of the skin had markedly changed. It appeared so clean, new, and rather different from the appearance of the rest of the foot. I was truly amazed at the total regeneration of my foot problem. I believe that a compromised immune system is at the root of the problem.

To test out this hypothesis, I refrained from spraying my foot to see if the condition would return. After 3 or 4 days, the itching and raw redness did indeed return, necessitating more applications of urine.

This testimony is being written in early July, and at this point, I am totally convinced of the effectiveness of urine application for skin problems. The infection always reappears if I do not make at least two appications daily, however, with conscientious applications, I have a seemingly normal foot with no chafing, redness, itching, and breaking.

I have shared this experience with my doctor who simply said, "I can't argue with success. Continue doing your low-cost, unconventional therapy (!)."

I am presently looking forward to the opportunity of taking in my urine once I feel I can put my medications aside and detoxify my body. I am presently researching the health benefits attributed to the drinking of one's urine, feeling that it must also be a truly wonderful spiritual experience with the miracle we call our body.

Sincerely yours,

Mr. Q. from New York

A note from the authors: Since we received this testimony, Mr. Q. has begun drinking his urine, and reported that his foot is completely healed. We are still collecting data on him and his AIDS condition.

Dear Doctor,

The reason I started using urine therapy is because I was sick. I was sick with diarrhea, abdominal and intestinal pain, a rash that eventually spread to both arms and legs, on my back, neck, head and face. This rash was extremely itchy (especially at night) and oozed a clear liquid when itched.

I have been to four doctors in almost three years for the same symptoms mentioned above; two holistic doctors (be very aware of doctors who claim to be so called "holistic", if they treat you with only drugs —FIRE THEM— they are not remotely close to being "holistic") and two general practicioners, who were in my opinion ignorant of all facts concerning the "Art of Healing", be especially aware of these practitioners.

Now my dear friends I had a question to ask myself and then a choice to make. The question was do I go to another doctor or do I trust my own intuition? The choice I made was to heal myself. I made the choice because I felt confident in my own knowledge of what was happening to my body. I had an open mind to alternative ways of healing my body. When I had an open mind urine therapy was introduced to me.

At first I wasn't impressed at all. Then two weeks later I found myself drinking my own urine and rubbing it on the infected areas of my body. Now listen to this my friends. Within four days of fasting (only drinking urine and water) and rubbing urine on my skin the symptoms mentioned earlier were disappearing rapidly. To this day one month later the diarrhea has stopped. The rash has almost gone away (there is no oozing of clear liquid anymore). Very little gas, and the abdominal pain have disappeared. I was in amazement and very pleased with my discovery of urine therapy.

Now let me be frank with you; the symptoms have not

gone away completely. I feel for two reasons: 1) I have not fasted long enough on only urine and water and 2) YOU MUST BE VERY AWARE OF THE FOODS YOU EAT —NO DENATURALIZED PROCESSED FOODS!!!!! I believe in this very strongly for when I eat these foods my symptoms flare up. So I know it is the foods I eat.

Urine therapy is a process. If you do not succeed fully the first time try and try again.

I am very grateful to have found urine therapy. I believe in urine therapy. It is FREE and it just may save your life.

With Universal Love,

Ronald E. from California

Dear Doctor,

In the summer of 1983, after extensive examinations, because of back pain, they found cancer in my spine. I had radiation treatments and the pain subsided. After that I treated myself by natural means. I injected myself with "Iscador" which gave me positive results.

In January 1986 I became sick again. I thought I had the flu because of the high fever, so I went to the local medical doctor. On examination he found a swollen liver. We did an ultrasound examination, and the doctor diagnosed Metastatic Cancer of the liver. They gave me pain killers, told me there was nothing they could do, and sent me home to die.

After the initial shock, I decided to find myself a doctor who thinks more positively. I found a homeopath who treated me with bioradiation. This gave me an increase in energy.

In November 1986 my condition worsened. I had hepatitis with high fever and intense pain. I was feeling very weak.

My last hope was urine therapy. I began drinking the "water of life". I drank only my first morning urine. By the 5th day I felt more energetic. By the 10th day I returned to the doctor. He could not believe I was still alive.

I drink my urine every morning to this day. I have to say that as of June 1987 my liver is again slightly swollen and my body itches all over, but I do not have any pain. I feel very positive.

Sincerely,

Mrs. E., Switzerland

"One day, I would have to tell the whole world about real healing"

UROPATHY (therapy — using urine), or the drinking of your own waters, came into my life in 1979. Two different friends gave me books on this subject on the same day. I could not wait to try it out. I found it easy to do. I read both books avidly, the "Water of Life" by John W. Armstrong and "Shiumbu Kalpa" by Arthur Lincoln Pauls, D.O. I was a believer from that very day of hearing the esoteric teachings. I did it every morning and also told people who were sickly and needed healing. It did not matter if they did it or believed it. I felt better about giving it away. I used it on my body when I had cuts or scratches, on a motorcycle burn, and on sunburns. All healed in a remarkably fast time. It even made my skin smooth and soft. It also is said, that it stops the aging process!

Then in June 1983 I was in a motorcycle accident, breaking my arm in three places, scraping the skin on my shoulder, arm, trunk, and leg. One side of my body was road burned several layers deep. Also, my sunglasses had to be pulled from my head. I had no eyebrow left. The plastic surgeon who stitched my head up was amazed by my rapid healing and did not understand it. I had no insurance so I went home to heal myself; broken arm and all. I could not walk upright. I did not take pain pills or any other medication. All I had for healing was my own urine. I applied it all over the open wounds. I never had a scab. My healing was from inside out. The body filled in from the bone to the muscles, and finally pink smooth skin. The regeneration on my head and eyebrow cannot be noticed today. I was back at work within one month. Many believe things happen for a reason. Yes, I was a believer before the accident, but after seeing myself heal so quickly, I knew that one day I would have to tell the whole world about real healing. The more I read and learned about this ancient healing practice, the more I realized that the world needs to know this truth today, especially with Cancer and AIDS facing our lives, and our children's lives. We must wake up to reality and cast away what is false. *Whatever is known to oneself, be gradually taught to others and many be made wise.* May you see this with the love that it is given.

With Universal Love,

M. from Florida

Dear World,

My experience with urine-therapy has been 2-fold. I was able to solve a yeast infection, relieve a chronic constipation problem, and began my menstrual flow after a 3 year ceasation.

Metaphysically, I began to "open" at an accelerated rate. Upon the eve of the first time I drank my water, I fill into a deep sleep in which I had a very significant out-of-body experience. I began to notice increased clairvoyance and clairaudience. I began to channel verbally as well as through automatic handwriting. Past life memories were activated, and I was able to see "Spirit-lights" (white sparkling dancing lights in the air). As time went on other colors began to be visible. I was given the gift of touch-healing and much, much more!

My experience has been wonderful! I believe in urine-therapy on every level. It is a God-sent gift to humanity for the resolution of dissension between mind, body and spirit.

Ms. L.J.M.
From Milwaukee, Wis.

Dear Margie,

I first heard of urine-therapy through your sister. We had been discussing how her vericous veins were so bad and how she put urine on them and they faded away within a few weeks. I had a skin condition where I was getting huge cyst like bumps all over my face and neck. She told me this therapy could help me.

I had already been to numerous medical doctors and had tried countless creams and medications which never helped. The doctors told me they were sebaceous cysts. I immediately started to apply urine to my face and throat. By the end of the one week the cysts were gone except for the largest one, which is now about the size of a pea. I have been using urine topically for two months and I plan on continuing this therapy for my skin disorder, as well as for my other health problems. I feel that urine is very beneficial as a healing agent.

                Sincerely,

                Diane from Florida

Dear Margie,

I am writing this in regard to your article in the Mighty Natural Directory about urine-therapy.

I was in India in 1968. I had a hysterectomy and was given a blood transfusion at that time. I used to be as healthy as a horse. In 1971 my husband died of a heart attack. He was only 47. I was left with the responsibility of taking care of my son, age 18, a daughter, age 14, and another daughter, age 12.

In 1973 I became totally bed-ridden I went to the best doctors in town and tried all kinds of treatment like Allopathy, Homeopathy, and Ayurvedic. My body did not respond to any of these methods; it could not absorb any medicine. My face would swell up, then my arms and legs, and I would be in utter pain wherever the swelling was.

Doctors could not diagnose what was wrong with me. I was sure I was dying and I had no appetite for six months. I was praying to God to spare my life otherwise my children would be left as orphans. An old friend of mine from Bombay came to visit me in Delhi and was shocked to see my condition and I started crying. She was completely undisturbed and asked, "why didn't you write to me about your health?" I said, "What can you do? You are no doctor." She gave me a thin book on urine-therapy and told me to read it. I finished reading it and was full of hope. Immediately I started following the instructions given in the book. Believe it or not in just three days I regained my appetite and my strength. I was so full of energy; I walked a mile and was not tired at all. I believe urine-therapy saved my life. I have not lost my appetite or my energy or fallen sick again to this day.

    Sincerely,

    Sara from Florida

Below are four testimonials of people who Sara had helped by telling them of urine-therapy.

I am a rich widow with one daughter, age 35, who is an engineer. I had developed some disease on my toes of my left foot. I went to the hospital and they gave me some ointment, but no improvement. It was diagnosed as leprosy. Then I met Sara and she told me to soak my foot in my own urine. In eight days my toes were as good as new. I went to the hospital again for a check up, they gave me a clean bill of health and asked me what I did. I told them I prayed to God. Even now my daughter does not know that I ever had leprosy, otherwise she would have admitted me in a hospital with the best of intentions and I probable would never have come back to see my home again.

    Sheila,
    from Bombay, India

In 1975, I had an irritation on the wrist of my right arm. I tried all kinds of ointments and salves. The rash would go completely away then come back again much worse. I had spent a fortune on it without any permanent results. When I met Sara, she told me to soak a handkerchief soaked in my own urine and tie it around my wrist for three days. To be sure I did it for eight days. My wrist cleared up and the disorder has not come back since then.

    Dana from Florida

I was aspiring to join a group of monks, but I had asthma and I smoked cigarrettes.

The group would not accept me because smoking was considered to be against the rules of spiritual training. I was ashamed of myself and felt very miserable. Then I met Sara and she instructed me on how to cure my asthma. I used urine-therapy, and in three days I stopped smoking completely and joined the group.

> Dharmanand
> from Delhi, India

I was suffering from stomach problems for two years. I had a constant stomach ache. I tried conventional medical treatment, herbs and teas, but no improvement. After Sara told me about urine-therapy, I began drinking my urine at once. Since then I have had no problems with my stomach or digestion.

> Nancy from Florida

Dear Margie.

To be honest, one of the main reasons I started with urine-therapy was financial. I was always one to try new natural compounds for healing. Afterall, once you go on a search to understand and listen to your body-mind-spirit sensitivities, there's a yearning for your balance and desire to alleviate all pain. In the past, I've often felt much confusion with all the choices of what to take, and how expensive it all is. "Why can't it be simple", I asked myself.

I feel my discovering of urine-therapy was no accident and probably the biggest blessing of my life. So far, within just the first five weeks, many skin irritations and small lumps that were under my arms for over a year are disappearing before my very eyes! My general appearance is more youthful and the amount of energy and stamina of my body has increased. I am also sensing that I am less judgemental of myself.

There's something very powerful going on in a deeper

sense. The only way to describe this is I'm feeling more psychic awareness. I'm taking hold of my life and am being guided toward real focusing.

        Susie
        from Miami, Florida

CONCLUSION

Based on all metaphysical and scientific evidence supporting UROPATHY, one cannot deny validity of this therapy.

UROPATHY is a daily, universal practice that only those who wish to avoid global peace and self-love, and the evolution of both will refuse.

It was used and described in every major religion, in Brotherhoods and sacred organizations. Now is the dawning of the New Age and mankind is ready to accept this truth.

UROPATHY has been successfully used on practically all maladies known to mankind. We believe AIDS will not be an exception to these statistics.

UROPATHY is the answer to the frustration in the AIDS community. AIDS will AID us to accept the Water of Life and restore it to be an integral part of our lives.

Thousands of terminally ill patients who are left hopeless can again be optimistic.

People need the freedom to decide what kind of healthcare they prefer. Whether it be the conservative medical route or an alternative method of healing, the choice should be left to the patient. We need to keep the freedom that our founding fathers intended us to have.

Judge Cooley of the U.S. Supreme Court said, "No right is held more sacred or is more carefully guarded by the common law, than the right of every individual to the possession and control of his/her own person."

Thomas Jefferson, writer of the U.S. Constitution, taught that "liberty in all essential needs, is not a privilege granted by Government, but an inherent right possessed by all men." The major function of the governments is to secure and enforce these human rights, not to violate them to satisfy medical dogmas and economic interests.

We are doing this work because we believe in the power within and that this truth must be revealed today.

There was a papyrus given to Dr. Bartnett with a calender of 1987 on it, it has Egyptian heiroglyphics that convey an important message. Dr. Bartnett has been well educated in Egyptian philosophy and was able to translate this papyrus. We would like to share it with you and end this publication with this beautiful translation.

May you find your inner-self, fill it with peace and love, and make the Water of Life an integral part of your existence.

"Blessed are those who are blind, but can see."

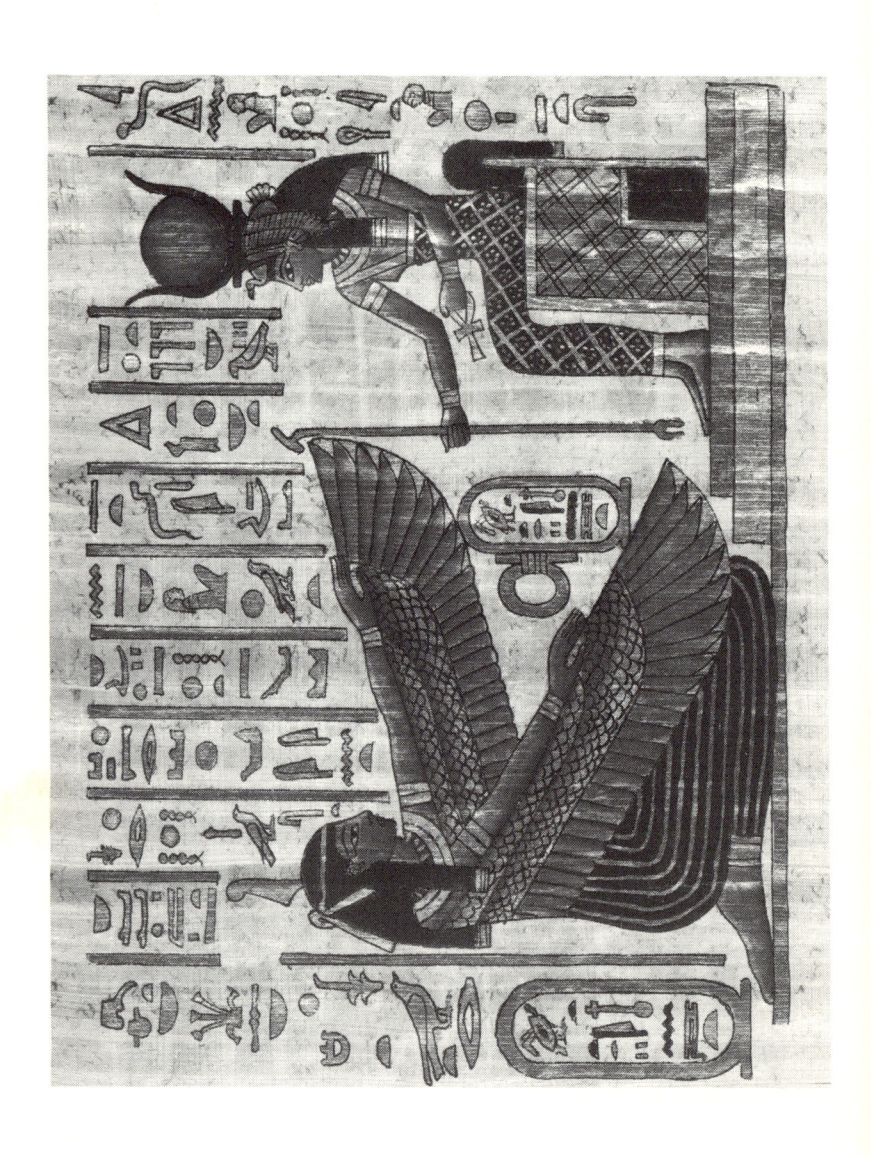

PAPYRUS TRANSLATION

The water of life is given to you, drink it and wash your body with it.

It is given to you for your spirit, mind, and body-for the man and woman inside of you.

The water of life is given to us to make us whole-oneness in ourselves.

It increases the ability of the hidden senses. It gives one courage, strength and freedom-freedom from fears and attachments.

The water of life will enable men and women to live together as one-in this world and in the world to come, making both worlds into one place.

The water of life will create a civilization far superior to the one existing. Noble character traits will be it's sign.

This civilization will guide the sciences and the arts-it will guide the spirit, mind, and body for further growth and increased wisdom.

It will give birth to the unity of both worlds.

The water of life will increase your love and knowledge-it makes you more whole.

It will help you to be what you are-a perfect creation.

Isis, the servant of mankind and mediator of the idea of creation, is giving the key of higher living.

With spirit, mind, and body, we have to guide men and women with wisdom similar to that of a priest, teaching the water of life and the life principles - for this world & the world to come.

SUGGESTED RESOURCES

Author	Name of Book
Airola	*How to Get Well*
Aivanhov	*The Mysteries of Yesod* **Vol. 7**
Allegro	*Dead Sea Scrolls and the Christian Myth*
DeRohan	*Right Use of Will*
Dinicin	*Book of Herbs*
Fankhauser	*The Power of Affirmation*
Foundation of Inner Peace	*Course in Miracles*
Gawain	*Creative Visualization*
Hay	*You Can Heal Your Life*
Hay	*Heal Your Body*
Jampolski	*Love is Letting Go of Fears*
Jampolski	*Teach only love*
Kloss	*Back to Eden*

Mindell	*Vitamin Bible*
Porvati	*Hygieia: A Woman's Herbal*
Parker/Roman	*Opening to Channel*
Prophet	*St. Germain on Alchemy*
Tierra	*The Way of Herbs*
Treben	*Health Through God's Pharmacy*
Yogananda	*Autobiography of a Yogy*

Artist	**Name of Cassette Tape**
Hay	*Morning/Evening Meditation, Self Healing, AIDS - A Positive Approach, Cancer: Your Healing Power, Loving Yourself - Songs and Meditations.*
Kitaro	*Best of Kitaro, Silk Road, Kitaro Ki, Tunhuang.*
Deuter	*Ectacy, Celebration, Haleakala.*
Galway	*Song of the Seashore.*
Marie	*Unicorn's Dream*
Vollenweinder	*Caverna Magica, Behind the Gardens, White Winds, Sun Singer.*

Anyone interested in the forthcoming cassette tapes that will assist you in making UROPATHY and integral part of your life and containing soothing meditative background music with self-reading positive affirmations to help break through the mental barriers and introduce you to UROPATHY should inquire through the **Water of Life Institute.**

BIBLIOGRAPHY

AIDS: The Mistery and the Solution *by Allen Cantwell,* **Aries Rising Press, 1983.**

AIDS, Cancer and the Medical Establishment *by Raymond Brown, M.D.,* **Aries Rising Press, Los Angeles, 1986.**

The Cancer Cure That Worked! *by Lynes and Crane,* **Marcus Books, 1987.**

The Dead Sea Scrolls and the Christian Myth *by John M. Allegro,* **Prometeus Books, 1984.**

The Holy Bible, *King James Edition,* **Thomas Nelson Publishers, 1979.**

The Lost Gospel of the Ages: Key to Immortality and Companion to the Holy Bible *by Hohn Christian Androgeus,* **Life Science Institute, 1978.**

Manav Mootra (Auto-Urine-Therapy) *by Raojubhai Manibhai Patel,* **(out of print).**

The Mysteries of Yesod *by Omraam Mikhael Aivanhov,* **Prosveta Publishers, 1982.**

Shivampu-Kalpa *by Dr. A.L. Pauls,* **(out of print).**

Dear friends,

We enjoy and look foreward to comments, suggestions, feedback, and inquiries concerning UROPATHY.

A quarterly publication in the near future will unite interested persons by sharing the information, stories, knowledge and experiences of people using UROPATHY. This will create a global bond, increasing peace and perpetuating healing for Mankind and Mother Earth.

For further information on UROPATHY, scheduled seminars, private consultations, and the book, **The Miracles of Urine-Therapy**, *please write to:*

The Water of Life Institute
P.O. Box 22-3543
Hollywood, Florida 33022-3543

Anyone wishing to make a donation to the Institute supporting the cause of eradicating dis-ease from the planet, your contribution and generosity will be deeply appreciated.

With Universal Love,

Dr. Beatrice Bartnett
Margie Adelman

Water of Life Institute
P.O. Box 22-3543
Hollywood, Florida 33022-3543

ORDER FORM

I would like to order _____ copies of the book **The Miracles of Urine-Therapy** (**$11.95** each). If Fla. resident add 6% sales tax.

Please send my order to:

NAME _____

ADDRESS _____

CITY _____

STATE _____ _____ ZIP _____

*Make all checks and money orders payable to: **Water of Life Institute**.
Shipment will be made upon receipt of your payment (in U.S. funds).
For postage and handling if shipped within the United States add $1.25 per book. Allow 2-3 weeks for delivery.
Foreign orders payable in U.S. funds. Canadian and Mexican orders add $2.00 in addition to U.S. postage, other foreign orders enclose $7.50 for shipping plus U.S. Postage. Your order will be shipped surface rate unless special air fee arrangements are made. These prices are based upon the shipment of each book.
For priority mail, add $3.00 to the original postage fee. Priority mail will be shipped within 72 hours of receipt.